Siegfried Gursche, MH

W9-BNP-784

Coconut Oil

Discover the Key to Vibrant Health

The miracle oil for
- **heart disease**
- **diabetes**
- **weight loss**
- **cancer**
- **and more**

with delicious recipes

books
Alive

Summertown
Tennessee

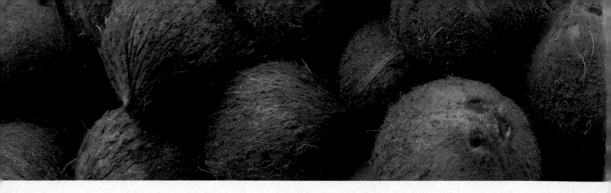

Contents

All About Coconut Oil

It is your constitutional right to educate yourself in health and medical knowledge, to seek helpful information and make use of it for your own benefit, and for that of your family. You are the one responsible for your health. In order to make decisions in all health matters, you must educate yourself. With this book and the guidance of a naturopath or alternative medical doctor, you will learn what is needed to achieve optimal health.

Those individuals currently taking pharmaceutical prescription drugs will want to talk to their health care professional about the negative effects that the drugs can have on herbal remedies and nutritional supplements, before combining them.

Healthy Recipes Using Coconut Oil and Coconut Flour

Note: Conversions in this book (from imperial to metric) are not exact. They have been rounded to the nearest measurement for convenience. Exact measurements are given in imperial. The recipes in this book are by no means to be taken as therapeutic. They simply promote the philosophy of both the author and *alive* books in relation to whole foods, health and nutrition, while incorporating the practical advice given by the author in the first section of the book.

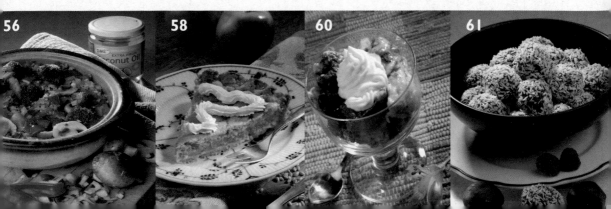

56   58   60   61

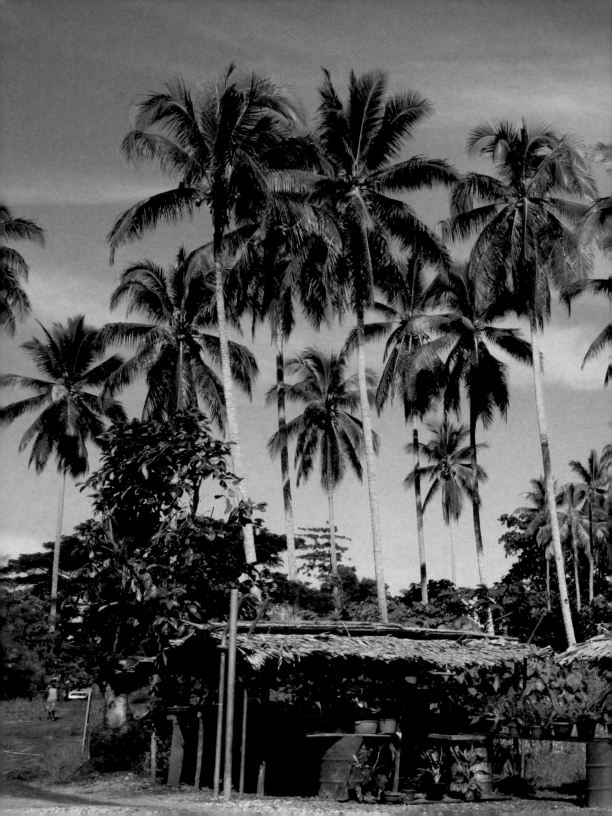

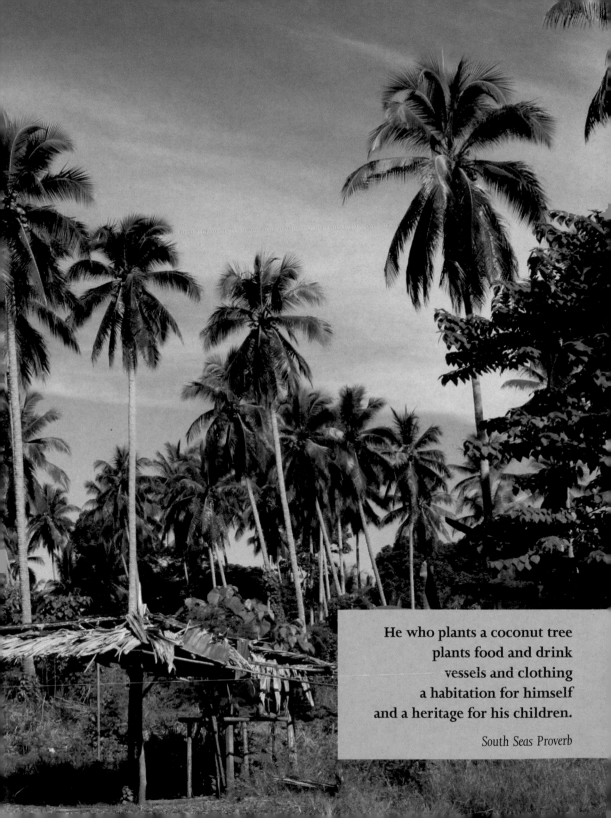

He who plants a coconut tree
plants food and drink
vessels and clothing
a habitation for himself
and a heritage for his children.

South Seas Proverb

Introduction . . . .

I must have been born with a keen interest in the natural world. When I think back to my childhood, where I grew up in a small German village close to nature, it seems those young years set me on a course to the career in the natural health industry that came decades later.

I remember my grandfather working a grain mill and running the general store full of bulk foods—this is where I had my first lessons about food. Since my father was an oil merchant, I also knew about good and bad fats at a very young age. I learned by watching the production process, and by eating them.

My father specialized in butter, handmade cheese, hazelnut and almond butters, freshly pressed flaxseed oil, and, yes, coconut oil. Coconut oil is not a new health food—it's older than I am! If I close my eyes, I can still smell the wonderful aroma of fresh, natural butters and oils my father produced. Once in a while my father would let me lick the parchment paper that had been used to cover them.

During that time, before World War II, the process of hydrogenation, the hardening of liquid oils, became a popular practice in the industry. My father sold only the best natural fats and oils. It wasn't until much later that researchers discovered that artifically hardened fats create unhealthy trans fats.

I am grateful for my healthy upbringing and the many opportunities I've had to learn about health throughout my life. Today I feel, in a way, that my purpose on Earth is to help as many people as possible to discover the health benefits of natural, fresh, nutritious foods, including unrefined virgin coconut oil.

In this guide I will help you to understand why high-quality coconut oil is so valuable for health. Please note that coconut oil and coconut butter are one and the same. Above room temperature the fat from coconuts appears as oil; at or below 24.5 degrees C (76 degrees F) it is more the consistency of soft butter.

No matter what you call it, coconut fat improves digestion and nutrient absorption; helps to fight infection and prevent degenerative disease; increases immunity; decreases inflammation; helps with weight loss; protects the liver and prostate; aids in healing skin conditions; is a safe beauty enhancer; is effective in the treatment of hypothyroidism and diabetes; and more.

It sounds too good to be true, I know. But it is true. Too bad most people don't know how powerfully nutritious and healing unrefined virgin coconut oil is. Most people, in fact, have been told that coconut oil is unhealthful and dangerous. I will explain how coconut oil got its bad reputation and why it is still demonized by many today, and I'll help you to rediscover the facts and truth about this healing oil.

I have written this book in layman's terms to help everyone understand the health benefits of high-quality coconut oil. With the proper information you, too, can follow in my father's footsteps by promoting natural goodness through optimal health. Finally, I want to help you put this information to practical use, so I will discuss ways of using coconut oil, and I'm sure you will enjoy the recipe section of this guide.

Coconut palms grow abundantly near water.

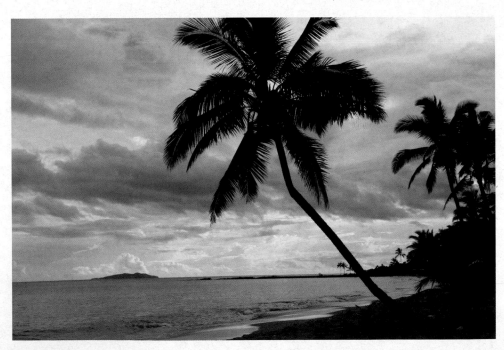

Do We Really Need Fat? . . . .

Before we talk more specifically about coconut oil, let's get a few things straight about fat in general. With the increase of obesity in Western civilization, people are hearing and asking more about fat, but are often left with even more questions.

What you know, or think you know, about good and bad fat depends on your source of information. For most people, large food manufacturers, with their seemingly unlimited marketing resources, are the ones spreading misinformation about fats. Large advertising dollars, continuously influencing our beliefs, easily overshadow the health-giving aspects of high-quality natural fats and other foods.

Adding to the confusion is the fact that many healthcare providers are just as confused as consumers, due to continuous advertising propaganda of the multinational food industry and half-truths from the governments it backs. Much of this information is supported by slanted or outdated scientific research.

Fatty functions

Of the fifty-one nutrients the human body requires for health, fat is the most misunderstood. With too little fat the body could not make use of fat-soluble vitamins A, D, E, and K. The membrane of each and every cell in the body is made up of fat, which provides both structure and flexibility. Most of the human brain is made up of different types of fat, including phospholipids and saturated and monounsaturated fats. Without fat the body cannot make hormones or the neurotransmitters that allow for physiological communication.

There's no doubt that the body needs more fat than most of us realize. Fat serves as an important backup fuel to our glucose, which we receive from carbohydrates. A healthy man carries about 20 percent of his weight as storage fat. A healthy woman carries 25 percent storage fat. The body can even make some of its own fat. Most of the body's stored fat is actually glucose that's been converted to fat for storage. In times of need this conversion is reversed and the fat becomes glucose again to be used for energy.

The essential fats we hear so much about these days cannot be produced by the body, which is why they are called essential. In other words, they are necessary for life but must be obtained through the diet since the body cannot make them from scratch. Without these essential fats, such as omega-3 and omega-6, the body cannot make what are called prostaglandins—hormone-like substances that activate many bodily functions and reactions.

It's true! We need fat to be healthy. Consuming a good amount of good fats will promote health. On the other hand, consuming too much of this nutrient will promote disease—especially if the fat being ingested is refined and denatured.

How Much Fat...and What Type? . . . .

One hundred years ago, when there were no refrigerators, people ate with the seasons. They enjoyed an abundance of carbohydrate-rich foods, such as berries and other fruit and vegetables, in the summer and early fall months. They put on pounds of fat as a result. In the winter, this stored fat was converted back to glucose fuel when food was scarce and calories were used for energy and to keep warm.

Today, of course, we have year-round access to food and can store food in our kitchens for weeks and months at a time. We no longer need to overeat, but many of us do. In addition, we have many poor carbohydrate food choices these days, including processed flour products, processed packaged foods, sugary drinks, and low-quality snacks. These "empty calories," as I like to call them, give us calories without any nutrients. We eat them and fill our stomachs and fill our fat stores, but leave our cells starving for nutrients. This is why when we eat processed foods we crave more processed foods and sugar. Whole foods, on the other hand, come with fibre and nutrients, including fat, to satisfy the body's needs.

As many people know, once fat has settled on the hips, it's hard to get rid of. Women, especially, have a difficult time losing fat due to their naturally higher fat ratio and regular hormonal fluctuations. My advice is to avoid processed carbohydrates altogether. Obtaining fat from a nutritious fat source, instead of from over-consumption of carbohydrates, is much healthier as natural fat is more easily metabolized or burned.

9

It's hard to visualize a gram of fat (which conatins 9 calories). If 33% of our daily diet is to come from fat (average 700 calories) we need to ingest the equivalent of about six pats of butter (10 g each), of course from a variety of sources.

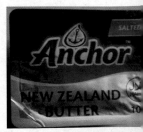

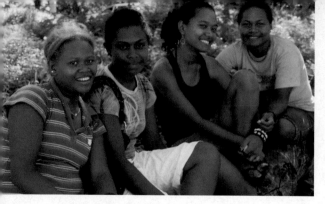

So, how much fat do we need? A healthy adult requires an estimated 70 grams (about 2½ ounces) of fat daily, but the quality is even more important than the quantity. Fat should come from good, natural, undamaged sources.

Low-fat opinions

Adoption of industrialized refined food by remote and tribal people has caused change of health trends in whole populations.

Since obesity has become common in our society, people have started to associate low-fat diets and diet products with health. However, eating low amounts of fat does not directly translate to lowering fat in the body. Research has shown that women who eat low-fat food products actually gain weight over time. I must even disagree with otherwise healthful, but low-in-fat, diets such as the McDougall diet plan.

John McDougall, founder and medical director of the nationally renowned McDougall Program, a ten-day residential program conducted at a luxury resort in Santa Rosa, California, recommends a low-fat diet plan. I agree with his suggestions to exclude white rice, coffee, and colas, but I disagree with his banning of foods such as butter, cheese, vegetable oils, and eggs. When these are of high quality and eaten in proper amounts, they promote health and even weight loss.

McDougall's weight loss plan teaches people to eat grains, vegetables, fruits, and beans. These are nutritious foods; however, in the long run I believe such a high-carbohydrate diet will leave people dissatisfied and looking for snacks. They will eat more carbohydrates and store them as fat, instead of eating high-quality fats that increase metabolism and help with weight maintenance and overall health. Others, such as Dr. Dean Ornish, have been criticized for their low-fat opinions as well. Dr. Ornish wrote several books promoting a low-fat diet, including *Dr. Dean Ornish's Program for Reversing Heart Disease* (Ivy Books 1995). I agree with his approach, which includes exercise and a vegetarian diet, but again feel that the fat intake he recommends is too low.

People who are deficient in fat may experience allergies, asthma, depression, hyperactivity, multiple sclerosis, rheumatoid arthritis, schizophrenia and, very commonly, skin disorders. I learned about the effects of fat deficiency from Dr. David Horrobin, a medical researcher, entrepreneur, author and editor, and pioneering contributor to the field of essential fatty acid research. I met him many times in his lab at the Efamol Research Institute in Kentville, Nova Scotia. His groundbreaking research and findings are supported by the practical experience of Elson M. Haas, MD, author of *Staying Healthy with Nutrition* (Celestial Arts 2006).

Fatty categories

From a molecular perspective, fats can be classified into three categories: saturated, monounsaturated, and polyunsaturated. Saturated fats have carbon chains that are saturated with hydrogen. In layman's terms, these fat chains have no open space for oxygen to hook onto. They are chemically stable fats. That's why saturated fats are solid at room temperature and last longer than unsaturated fats.

Unsaturated fats do have space for oxygen to hook onto. Monounsaturated fat chains have only one opening. They are not as stable as saturated fat, but are more stable than polyunsaturated ("poly" means "many") fat. Essential fatty acids fall into the polyunsaturated fat category. They are very chemically unstable. That's why we always store flaxseed oil, which is high in essential fatty acids, in the fridge and we never heat it.

As of late, we've learned even more about the makeup of fats. Within the above three categories are additional characteristics, or families, of fats. Some are short-chain, some medium-chain, and some long-chain. So, for example, a saturated fat may contain short-chain, medium-chain, and long-chain fatty acids. The same is true for monounsaturated and polyunsaturated fats. The short- and medium-chain fatty acids have a low melting point. The long-chain fatty acids have a higher melting point.

What Type of Fat is Virgin Coconut Oil?

Unrefined virgin coconut oil's many benefits can be explained, in part, by its unique composition. Unrefined virgin coconut oil is high in saturates, made up of mostly short and medium-chain fatty acids, and contains an extremely high amount of beneficial lauric acid.

Coconut oil's high saturated fatty acid content is the reason it is often incorrectly lumped into the "bad" fat category along with animal fat. However, the saturates in unrefined virgin coconut oil

Medium-Chain Fatty Acids in a Nutshell

- Coconut oil contains predominantly medium-chain fatty acids, also known as medium-chain triglycerides, which make it a much healthier oil than fats containing mostly long-chain fatty acids, such as animal fat.
- The medium-chain fatty acids in coconut oil are rapidly absorbed, then carried by the portal vein to the liver and converted into immediate energy, which means they are not stored, as long-chain fatty acids are.
- Medium-chain fatty acid molecules are small and can easily permeate cell membranes, while most other vegetable oils and animal fats consist of long chain fatty acids, which are larger.
- Medium-chain fatty acids are easily metabolized and do not require lipoproteins or special enzymes in order to be effectively utilized by the body. As mentioned above, medium-chain fatty acids are used as energy, while long-chain fatty acids are stored as fat.
- There is no danger of medium-chain fatty acids being stored in the arteries as long-chain fatty acids are.
- The medium-chain fatty acids in unrefined virgin coconut oil help to regulate thyroid function, stimulate metabolism (leading to weight loss), balance blood sugar level, increase energy, and promote overall health.

are plant-based and are not composed mainly of long-chain fatty acids, as is the case with animal saturates. Short- and medium-chain fatty acids behave differently in the body than long-chain fatty acids, such as those found in beef fat. The high amount of medium-chain and other saturated fats in unrefined virgin coconut oil is what makes the oil so stable, which means it is resistant to rancidity and safe for use as a food supplement and for cooking and baking.

Fatty Acid Composition of Virgin Coconut Oil

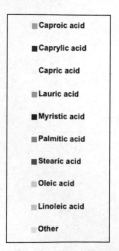

- Caproic acid
- Caprylic acid
- Capric acid
- Lauric acid
- Myristic acid
- Palmitic acid
- Stearic acid
- Oleic acid
- Linoleic acid
- Other

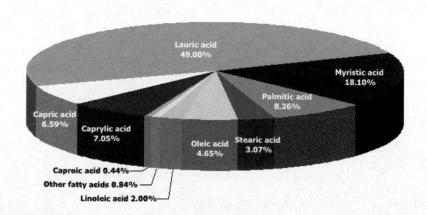

Lauric acid 49.00%
Myristic acid 18.10%
Palmitic acid 8.26%
Capric acid 6.59%
Caprylic acid 7.05%
Oleic acid 4.65%
Stearic acid 3.07%
Caproic acid 0.44%
Other fatty acids 0.84%
Linoleic acid 2.00%

The stability of high-quality coconut oil is one of the many reasons it promotes health (lower quality coconut oil, made from dried coconut flesh that has been refined, bleached, and deodorized, is disease-promoting). Due to its saturated fat content, virgin coconut oil in liquid form has the longest shelf life compared to any other oil, lasting up to three years. Coconut oil is best stored in solid form (at temperatures lower than 24.5 degrees C/76 degrees F), which will extend shelf life even further.

Fresh tropical fruit juice and coconut makes a well-rounded, satisfying, nutritious breakfast.

13

Aside from coconut oil's stability, up-to-date research tells us that medium-chain fatty acids are a burning, not a storing, fat, which means they actually help increase metabolism, aiding in weight loss and promoting health in a host of other ways.

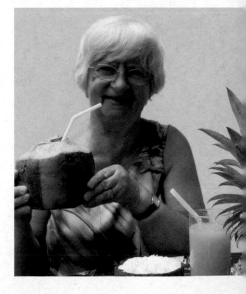

Yet another reason unrefined virgin coconut oil's composition is unique and beneficial to health is its very high content of lauric acid. Research tells us that lauric acid, a medium-chain fatty acid that is converted to monolaurin in the body, helps to lower LDL cholesterol and inactivates pathogens. Lauric acid is missing from our modern-day diet, but high-quality coconut oil is a safe, delicious way to benefit from this nutrient.

How Did Coconut Oil Get a Bad Reputation?

Coconut oil has been a part of healthful diets for thousands of years, consumed by those native to the tropics and even in non-tropical countries. Its reputation as a health-promoting oil has been known for centuries.

Prior to World War II, coconut oil was popular in North America, used widely in kitchens for hot food preparations, such as baking cookies and fabulous piecrusts. Restaurants used this stable oil to fry food, and it coated popcorn in the movie theatres. Despite this popularity, North Americans eventually came to think of coconut oil as dangerous and fattening.

Today, coconut oil has virtually disappeared except in the kitchens and restaurants of those who are "in the know" about fats and health. What happened? The answer is multi-faceted; however, the politics and economics of big food business played a key role.

During the war, Japanese forces occupied the Philippines, and the supply of coconut oil to the United States was interrupted. This led to an increased production of vegetable oil seeds, such as corn, sunflower, and soy, on North American farms. When the war was over, trade and commerce with the Philippines resumed and coconut oil once again became a desired commodity. North American vegetable oil producers were not happy to share the oil business.

Corn Products Company (now Corn Products International) and the American Soybean Association started a negative publicity campaign to convince the growing fast food industry and general public that unsaturated oils produced in the US were a better choice than coconut oil. Interestingly, the Center for Science in the Public Interest (CSPI), which today is regarded as a respected consumer advocate group, offered a loud voice and much support to this campaign. Despite much of their good work in other areas, CSPI continues to speak out against coconut oil today.

The new US vegetable oils were erroneously touted as heart healthy, and information about how cheap, refined, processed oils actually cause

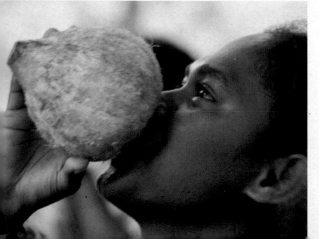

Coconut milk is a refreshing healthy drink.

heart disease was conveniently left out of the circulating information. Eventually, North Americans were brainwashed. At the same time, coconut oil was actively condemned, using seed oil industry dollars. Saturated fats were blamed for the epidemic rise in heart disease, which is just plain incorrect.

Saturated fat does not cause heart disease

It is a myth that saturated fats cause heart disease and a fallacy that polyunsaturated fats are heart healthy, according to Uffe Ravnskove, MD, PhD., a Danish independent researcher and member of various international scientific organizations. Dr. Ravnskove did extensive research that disproved the current, widely popularized lipid (fat) hypothesis used to explain the cause of heart disease. His findings have been accepted by professionals in Europe, while the North American and Canadian heart and stroke foundations ignore this important, up-to-date research. The English translation of his renowned book is called *The Cholesterol Myths: Exposing the Fallacy that Saturated Fat and Cholesterol Cause Heart Disease* (NewTrends Publishing 2000).

Dr. T. Rajamohan, professor at the Department of Biochemistry, University of Kerala, India, has human studies that clearly disprove the allegation against coconut oil. In one of his studies, each of the 258 participants consumed an average of 38 grams of coconut oil per day. The results indicated that coconut oil consumption does not cause an increase in LDL cholesterol, but does increase beneficial HDL cholesterol.

World-renowned nutritionist and biochemist Mary G. Enig, PhD, co-founder and vice president of the Weston A. Price Foundation, agrees. She suggests that complex ingredients in coconut oil, such as lauric acid, reduce LDL and improve HDL cholesterol. Enig has widely stated: "The problems for coconut oil started four decades ago when researchers fed animals hydrogenated coconut oil that was purposely altered to make it completely devoid of any essential fatty acids . . . The animals fed the hydrogenated coconut oil (as the only fat source) naturally became essential fatty acid-deficient; their serum cholesterol increased." She points out that essential fatty acid deficiency always produces an increase in serum cholesterol levels. The same effect is seen with any type of highly hydrogenated oils, not just hydrogenated coconut oil.

High Heat Damages Fat

When high heat is applied to oils, especially polyunsaturated fats, damaged fat molecules result. These heat-damaged molecules are damaging to the body when ingested. They increase the free radical damage that contributes to the development of degenerative diseases, such as cancer and heart disease.

Unrefined virgin coconut oil is heat-stable with a smoke point of 230 degrees C (446 degrees F)—the highest of any unrefined vegetable fat. As a comparison, the smoke point of olive oil is 190 degrees C (374 degrees F) and the smoke point of flaxseed oil is 112 degrees C (234 degrees F).

Enig strongly advises that heart disease is a complex illness with a number of causes, but insists that saturated fats and dietary cholesterol are not among them. I agree with her, and I'll say it again: Saturated fats do not cause heart disease, plain and simple. If they did, heart disease would not be new to this century. Historically, rural North Americans ate beef, pork, bacon, and eggs regularly, with no atherosclerosis, strokes, or heart attacks. Pointing a finger at saturated fats is not the answer.

If dietary fat really caused an increase in cholesterol and heart disease, low-fat and no-cholesterol diets would have lowered our epidemic rates of heart disease by now. However, heart disease remains the number one killer in the US, Canada, and in much of the Western world. Heat-treated, hydrogenated fats with trans fatty acids are largely responsible for this century's degenerative diseases. Contrary to popular belief, low-fat diets actually increase fat levels in the blood, as proven by researchers A.H. Lichtenstein and L. Van Horn. In the long run, high triglyceride (fat) levels lead to insulin resistance, which is a factor in obesity, type 2 diabetes, and heart disease.

One of the first studies conducted on coconut oil, prior to World War II, was by Hans Kaunitz, who emigrated from Austria to Manila to teach medicine at the University of the Philippines. His research clearly showed that increased cholesterol and clogged arteries only occurred in lab animals when they were fed hydrogenated coconut oil with no essential fatty acids. When consuming high-quality coconut oil they were healthy, just like the people native to the tropics.

We've known, scientifically, for more than six decades that unrefined virgin coconut oil promotes health. On the other hand, there is no clear-cut evidence, scientific or otherwise, that

16

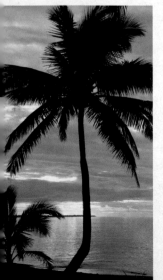

In the Phillippines they call the palm "Tree of Life."

cholesterol causes heart disease. David Rowland, PhD, founder of the Canadian Nutrition Institute and education director of the Edison Institute of Nutrition, reported years ago that cholesterol levels rise more in response to dietary sugars, caffeine, and alcohol than they do to either dietary fats or the consumption of cholesterol. In any case, natural virgin coconut oil is free of cholesterol.

The answer to this vicious cycle of disease can only be answered by returning to a diet of natural, unprocessed foods, high in nutrients and fibre. Common sense, and empirical evidence gathered by Dr. Weston-Price during his travels and studies among Polynesians and other coconut-consuming tribes in the 1970s, tells us that natural virgin coconut oil does not cause heart disease or any other degenerative diseases. The opposite is true: It promotes health and prevents disease.

Propaganda prevails

Interestingly, the hydrogenated coconut oil study that Enig cites as being so damaging to coconut oil's reputation was done just in time for the seed oil producers to use it in their campaign to blame heart disease on saturated fats. What this study really revealed is that once oils are manipulated and denatured, even a naturally good fat can be turned into a bad one. However, the seed oil industry and CSPI reported the results in a slanted fashion, without taking into consideration that any modified, hydrogenated oil is dangerous.

Unfortunately, the poorer tropical oil industries of Indonesia, India, and the Philippines could not afford to counter the twisted science and negative propaganda spread by those in the US in the late 1980s. Their expensive campaign has paid off for decades now. Many people who are sincerely interested in truthful information and natural health have been fooled.

History has proven that propaganda works. When told often enough, the public will accept and believe lies and untruths and act accordingly, often without question or looking to alternative sources.

As reported in the Philippine journal *Coconut Today* (November 2005), the latest threat to coconut oil,

The #1 industry on the Solomon Islands is the production and export of copra for the commercial oil and margarine manufacturers.

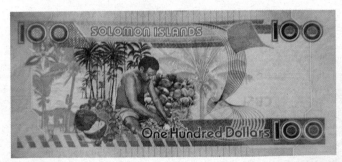

17

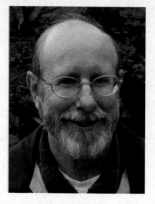

Dr. Bruce Fife, ND, Director of the Coconut Research Centre, calls virgin coconut oil "the healthiest oil on earth."

in relation to the smear campaign perpetuated by the US-based oilseed companies, is a new regulation by Health Canada and the US Food and Drug Administration. As of January 1, 2006, food nutrition labels require the listing of trans fats together with saturated fats, which implies that both of these fats contribute to the development of disease. No consideration is made for saturated fat consisting of medium-chain fatty acids, such as the good saturates in coconut oil. Unrefined virgin coconut oil is naturally trans fat-free.

With so much effort to demonize coconut oil, many have missed out on years of health benefits. In fact, the benefits of consuming unrefined virgin coconut oil are so many that they seem miraculous.

Miraculous Health Benefits of Coconut Oil

As an increasing amount of people discover the healthful and healing qualities of high-quality coconut oil, the list of benefits continues to grow. Most modern-day scientists are just beginning to understand what indigenous people of the tropics have known for centuries. Unrefined virgin coconut oil

- Improves nutrient absorption
- Helps prevent osteoporosis
- Boosts energy
- Increases metabolism
- Aids in weight loss
- Treats digestive disorders
- Treats candidiasis
- Protects against bacterial and viral infection
- Treats herpes complex virus
- Increases immunity
- Helps protect the liver
- Helps prevent cardiovascular disease
- Helps prevent cancer
- Decreases inflammation
- Helps prevent hypoglycemia
- Treats enlarged prostate
- Heals skin conditions
- Protects and moisturizes skin
- Heals skin burns
- Increases hair health
- And more.

The Healthiest Oil on Earth

Many natural health experts, including Bruce Fife, PhD, ND, CN, and director of the nonprofit Coconut Oil Research Centre, call coconut oil the healthiest oil on earth. High-quality coconut oil is known in the natural health industry as a functional food. That is, it naturally offers significant healing and health-promoting benefits—and with no side effects!

Thanks in large part to the modern research of the late Conrado S. Dayrit, we have some idea of just how miraculous coconut oil is for health and healing. The list of ways coconut oil promotes health is seemingly endless and I won't be able to do it justice in this book. But let's take a closer look at some of the ways coconut oil can play a role in health, healing, and disease prevention. First we'll look at how coconut oil promotes health in many general ways, then I'll discuss some of the many specific diseases, conditions, and ailments that can be improved with coconut oil.

Increase nutrient absorption

One benefit of high-quality coconut oil that can improve everyone's health is increased nutrient absorption. Increased nutrient absorption leads to increased nourishment of cells and increased health. As published in the *American Journal of Clinical Nutrition* (September 1996), researchers at the University of Iowa found that when babies were fed formula rich in coconut oil they showed improved absorption of fats and minerals.

Those working to regain health may especially benefit from the improved nutrient absorption that results from consuming coconut oil. People concerned about osteoporosis, for example, may benefit from consuming coconut oil since it increases mineral absorption to build and strengthen bones.

Increase energy

For those who feel fatigued, or suffer from chronic fatigue, two teaspoons of unrefined virgin coconut oil in the morning and one teaspoon in the afternoon will increase energy. Coconut oil does not give the jolt of energy that coffee does, which incidentally wears out the adrenal glands, leading to increased fatigue over the long run. Instead it offers a more subtle, sustaining energy. Try it for four to six weeks and notice the effects.

Medium-chain fatty acids, of which coconut oil is mostly composed, are a hot topic in the field of sports nutrition because they represent an immediate source of energy. Medium-chain fatty acids bypass the longer process of digestion and assimilation that all other fats must go through before being either utilized or stored as backup energy. Medium-chain fatty acids are assimilated quickly and easily, and are therefore burned, not stored, in the body.

Aid digestion

Digestive disorders are common in today's society. Since unrefined virgin coconut oil is easy to digest, improves nutrient absorption, protects from infection, and decreases inflammation, it is an excellent choice for those with intestinal conditions.

Research shows, for example, that the anti-inflammatory properties of coconut oil help to reduce the irritation that accompanies Crohn's disease. The bacteria and viruses that are often cited as contributing factors or causes of ulcerative conditions may be fought with the antimicrobial properties present in coconut oil. In addition, those with gallbladder problems, or difficulty digesting fats, may benefit from consuming coconut oil since it does not require pancreatic enzymes or bile for its breakdown and metabolism.

Fight infection

The powerful antifungal and antimicrobial properties in coconut oil are effective in treating a wide range of bacteria, fungi and viruses, including herpes simplex. Both the lauric and capric acids in coconut oil are beneficial in treating intestinal yeast infections such as candidiasis.

In the body, lauric acid is converted into monolaurin, which appears to inactivate or destroy lipid enveloped viruses, such as HIV, measles, herpes simplex virus, influenza, and rubella. While antibiotics do nothing to prevent or treat viruses, coconut oil may help to do both. Reports from the Philippines say that people, when feeling the onslaught of flu, drink half a cup of coconut oil for an immediate cure.

According to researcher Stephen Byrnes, PhD, ND, RNCP, author of the critically acclaimed book *Overcoming AIDS with Natural Medicine* (Ecclesia Life Mana 1997), the first clinical trial involving monolaurin has recently been completed in the Philippines. The results indicate a greater than 50 percent reduced viral load in subjects. The study also showed that the patients using coconut oil showed better results than those simply taking monolaurin supplements.

Boost immunity

The high content of antimicrobial lipids and lauric, capric, and caprylic acids in unrefined virgin coconut oil have been shown to benefit the immune system. The immune system is the control center for overall health and defense against disease. Dr. Enig's research suggests that those who have compromised immunity should eat approximately 25 grams of lauric acid per day, which is equivalent to about four tablespoons of coconut oil.

If you tend to catch every cold that's going around, you will benefit from supplementing your diet with virgin coconut oil. Many people living with HIV, for example, have reported a decrease in their viral load and improved overall health as a result of including coconut in their diets.

Decrease inflammation

Inflammation is a much-researched subject today, as scientists speculate that it is a major contributing factor to the development of disease. While anti-inflammatory drugs simply mask disease symptoms and interrupt the natural healing process, coconut oil may help reduce the inflammation naturally, to aid healing. A study from the Institute of Human Nutrition at the University of Southampton, UK, published in the journal Immunology (March 1999), concluded that coconut oil may be useful in the treatment of both acute and chronic inflammation and inflammatory diseases, including heart disease.

Prevent degenerative disease

According to Dr. Dayrit, coconut oil aids in the prevention of cardiovascular disease and cancer because it helps to protect the blood from free radical damage (Philippine Journal of Cardiology 2003). Natural, unrefined coconut oil does not become rancid as easily as other fats and is not toxic

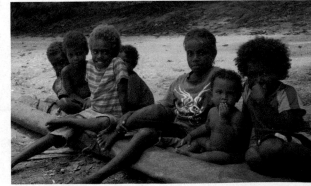

Healthy children on the Solomon Islands, where very few people suffer from degenerative diseases.

due to processing procedures, thus sparing consumers from toxicity and free radical damage. In addition, coconut oil may aid the body in eliminating disease-causing germs, which relieves stress on the immune system. This allows the white blood cells to function more efficiently, which helps to eliminate cancerous cells and prevent development of cancer.

Dayrit's Discoveries

When I first heard about the tremendous findings Conrado S. Dayrit, MD, FACC, FPCC, FPCP, of the National Academy of Science and Technology, had with coconut oil, I knew I had to speak with him. I found the emeritus professor at the University Hospital in Manila, still academically active at his then age of 87. Our telephone conversation turned out to be a lengthy one, and I gained a high respect for his clinical work. During his time at the Victor R. Potenciano Medical Center in Manila, Dr. Dayrit directed the cardiology department. It was there that he discovered and confirmed that unrefined virgin coconut oil is a heart-friendly oil. I was even more amazed to hear about the positive findings in his first formal study of coconut oil as an effective treatment of HIV/AIDS. It is with great thanks and respect that I say goodbye to the great researcher and humanitarian Dr. Dayrit. He passed away in November 2007.

Coconut Treats Specific Conditions

Dayrit, Fife, and other experts recommend a host of ways coconut oil can both cure disease and prevent it, including degenerative diseases such as cancer, heart disease, and type 2 diabetes. People interested in natural beauty care love coconut oil. Research also shows it may be helpful in the treating enlarged prostate, digestive disorders, hypothyroidism, weight loss, skin disorders, and even HIV/AIDS. Both empirical evidence and anecdotal success stories are circulating like wildfire.

Conrado Dayrit, MD, wrote the book The Truth about Coconut Oil: The Drugstore in a Bottle

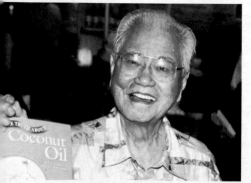

Cancer

Statistics tell us that one out of every three people in the Western world will develop some form of cancer in their lifetime. Cancer is a disease that reaches into every family. We all know situations where the treatment for cancer has been more painful and debilitating than the disease itself. It's not surprising that a growing number of people are exploring alternative ways to decrease their risk.

As mentioned earlier, coconut oil offers protection from the free radical damage that contributes to the development of degenerative diseases, including cancer. Another very important way coconut oil helps to prevent cancer is through boosting the immune system.

It wasn't very long ago that science discovered the fact that we all carry cancer cells—even the healthiest among us. The trouble starts when the immune system becomes incapable of destroying these malignant cells. That's when cancer develops. Knowing this, there is much we can do to lower our risk of developing cancer.

Low immunity and high acidity, both of which increase risk of cancer development, result from poor diet and lifestyle choices and habits. Overconsumption of animal proteins, sugar, and processed foods suppresses immunity and creates acidity. Leading a stressful life will have the same negative effects. When it comes to fats, processed oils increase cancer risk in two ways—they lower immunity by causing inflammation in the body, and they cause free radical damage.

Since a strong, healthy immune system can keep cancer cells in check, it makes sense to invest in a high-quality fat that supports immunity. Unrefined virgin coconut oil is safe to cook with and does the opposite of refined oils. It decreases inflammation and increases immunity.

In one of my conversations with Dr. Dayrit, I asked him why there hadn't been a large medical study to see whether unrefined virgin coconut oil was as effective against cancer as some people were finding. He explained that since coconut oil and its derivatives are natural products they cannot be patented. With no patent potential the large companies that fund such research are not interested because the research results cannot be protected for any return in investment. Sad, but true. Cancer is big business today.

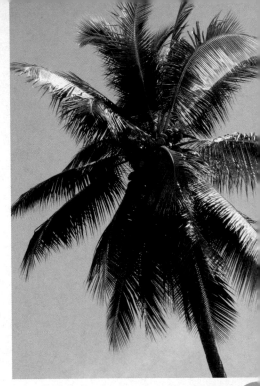

Hundreds of different species of coconut palms grow in equatorial countries around the world.

Candida

The yeast overgrowth infection known as candidiasis, or candida, is a difficult one to heal. It is caused by an overgrowth of an unfriendly bacteria called Candida albicans, and develops when friendly lactic-acid bacteria are depleted in the gut, either by a poor diet high in sugary and processed foods or as a result of prescription drugs, especially antibiotics.

Antibiotics are very good at killing off the harmful bacteria they are designed to kill. Unfortunately, they also kill the friendly bacteria, too. Yeast such as the species C. albicans are not affected by antibiotics and, therefore, are free to flourish once there are no friendly bacteria to keep them in check. Such a yeast imbalance results in infection that compromises the immune system and overall health. Yeast infections plague more than half of all North American women and many men as well.

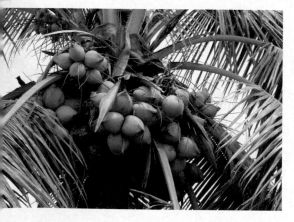

Dr. Renato M. Labadan coined the term "Coconut—The Philippines' Money Tree"

In the 1980s Jon J. Kabara, a professor of microbiology at Michigan State University, discovered that the lauric acid in coconut oil was the most potent antiviral, antibacterial, and antifungal agent of all fats and oils he had tested in his laboratory. According to his research, virgin coconut oil's lauric acid has the that coconut oil might do that. Since she owned a coconut plantation in Quezon province, she decided to retire there and make her own virgin coconut oil. She consumed as much as she could, mixing it with her food and beverages. Six months later she was feeling well and strong, with no signs or symptoms of her cancer. She was asked to return to the US for a follow-up. Surprised, the doctors told her that her cancer was "in remission." They asked her what she was taking; she answered, "Nothing but virgin coconut oil." She is back attending to her business ventures and recommends virgin coconut oil to all her friends. –Dr. Dayrit

Could Julie's previous chemotherapy have had a delayed effect? Dr. Dayrit felt this was extremely unlikely. He explained, "The cancer metastasized to the brain shortly after (perhaps even during) her chemotherapy. Chemotherapy stops the body's immune reaction." He speculates that the virgin coconut oil must have boosted Julie's immune system to put her cancer into a state of remission. The big question now is whether virgin coconut oil can result in a disappearance of cancer altogether and whether it can prevent cancer from developing in the first place.

ability to kill unfriendly yeast cells while keeping the friendly bacteria working.

Recent research backs up Kabara's findings. Findings from the University College Hospital, in Ibadan, Nigeria (*Journal of Medicinal Food* June 2007), show that virgin coconut oil is an effective antifungal agent in the treatment of yeast overgrowth. Researchers concluded that coconut oil should be recommended in the treatment of fungal infections, especially in view of emerging drug-resistant Candida species.

In the South Pacific, and elsewhere in the tropics, coconuts are part of the daily diet and yeast infection is practically unknown. In addition to effectively treating yeast overgrowth, coconut oil is helpful in other cases of bacterial infection, such as athlete's foot.

Diabetes

I cannot stress enough how powerfully beneficial unrefined virgin coconut oil is in the treatment of diabetes, for many reasons.

While eating foods high in carbohydrates, especially refined carbohydrates lacking fibre, results in a quick rush of glucose and rapid change in blood sugar levels in the body, coconut oil's high content of medium-chain fatty acids provides a ready source of energy without disrupting blood sugar levels. Steady blood sugar levels help to prevent hypoglycemia, a precursor to type 2 diabetes.

Because unrefined virgin coconut oil does not require pancreatic enzymes and does not raise blood sugar levels, it is a fat that diabetics can enjoy and benefit from. Coconut oil's ability to

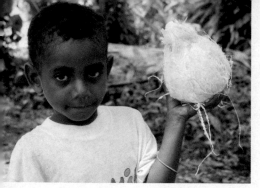

Where there are coconuts in the daily diet, there is reduced incidence of the chronic illnesses that plague Western society.

increase metabolic rate and aid in weight loss is also a benefit for those with type 2 diabetes.

According to Mike Foale, author of *The Coconut Odyssey* (Australian Centre for International Agricultural Research 2003), since coconut oil quickly converts to heat energy, it can be substituted for sugars as a ready source of energy without stimulating the release of insulin.

Eating naturally occurring fat (not trans fats or refined vegetable oils) has proven to be the most important method for ensuring fat loss and warding off diabetes. Fats from coconut oil, as well as fresh seeds, nuts, avocados, and fish, do not cause a spike in the fat-storing hormone insulin. This phenomenon has been proven many times.

Research at the Australian Centre for International Agriculture Research finds that extremes in blood sugar concentration are averted in people with diabetes if they consume a diet substituting coconut oil for sugars. A diet that includes coconut oil will also delay the development of the insulin resistance that triggers mature–onset diabetes in middle-aged people as well as younger, usually obese, individuals.

A study from the Department of Medicine, Safdarjang Hospital in New Delhi (*Journal of Indian Medical Association* October 1998), found ample research data to indicate that the sole use or excess intake of polyunsaturated vegetable oils is actually detrimental to health. It also found that switching to a combination of different types of fats, including traditional cooking fats like coconut oil, would actually reduce the risk of diseases including type 2 diabetes and heart disease.

Dr. Bruce Fife, who has written many books about coconut oil, including *The Coconut Oil Miracle* (Avery 2004), considers high-quality coconut oil one of the best foods for diabetics. He says, "Coconut oil has no adverse effect on blood sugar. When it is added to other foods it lowers the glycemic index of these foods and helps control blood sugar in diabetics." The glycemic index (GI) indicates the effect a food has on blood sugar. The lower a food is rated on the GI the better it is in terms of blood sugar stability. (However, the GI does not account for food quality. Ice cream, for example, is low on the GI but, as we know, is not a healthful food choice.) When we choose whole foods with their fibre intact, carbohydrates are digested at a slow enough rate to provide a steady release of glucose.

Heart disease

As discussed earlier, the medium-chain saturates in unrefined virgin coconut oil do not cause heart disease. Damaged fats and oils, along with other diet and lifestyle factors, are contributors. Refined oils, whether they are saturated, monounsaturated, or polyunsaturated, cause free radical damage in the body and inflammation in the arteries.

While the mainstream health authorities promote canola and other vegetable oils for heart health, natural health experts know that this information is incomplete. Since coconut oil is helpful in decreasing inflammation, it helps to prevent and treat heart disease. Also, unrefined virgin coconut oil and omega-3 oils are the only dietary oils known to reduce blood stickiness, which is beneficial for carrying more oxygen to the heart.

HIV/AIDS

Coconut oil is not only antifungal and antimicrobial, it is also antiviral. This makes it effective in treating viruses, including the flu and herpes simplex virus. Does this mean it can offer hope to the many people with HIV or AIDS? Yes, it does.

While antibiotics do nothing to prevent or treat viruses, virgin coconut oil may do both. Research by Dr. Dayrit in 2000 showed that both the lauric and capric acids in coconut oil are effective in killing HIV in lab cultures.

After lauric acid is converted to monolaurin in the body, it appears to inactivate or destroy lipid-enveloped viruses such as HIV, herpes simplex, chicken pox, shingles, and the common flu. Even the syncytial virus, a major cause of respiratory illness in young children, and the highly infectious rubella virus (German

Researchers are hopeful that coconut might provide an affordable cure for HIV/AIDS

measles), may be successfully treated with coconut oil.

Earlier, in 1998, Dayrit did the first clinical trial on HIV treatment with coconut oil using 15 infected people in the Philippines. The subjects, who had never received any treatment before, showed a greater than 50 percent reduced viral load. The study also showed that using coconut oil was more effective than simply supplementing with monolaurin. Since then, many people who are living with HIV have reported a decrease in their viral load and improved overall health after adding coconut oil to their treatment regime.

Hypothyroidism

The debilitating lack of energy that results from low thyroid function can be effectively treated with virgin coconut oil. According to Mike Foale, "The enhanced energy release, accompanied by a rise in body temperature attributed to the use of coconut, stimulates the thyroid gland, which governs the body's metabolism."

In addition to stimulating metabolism, coconut oil increases nutrient absorption, as mentioned earlier, which in turn leads to

Testimony: Coconut Oil Cures

Hello Mr. Gursche,

Thank you for the information on coconut oil. I have experienced some amazing changes in my life since I first started taking coconut oil. In the past, I suffered from high blood pressure, type 2 diabetes, and was a bit overweight.

Six months after I started the coconut oil regimen, my doctor determined that I was no longer diabetic. Today I take no diabetes medicine and have no signs of diabetes. Also, whenever my blood pressure is high, I find that taking a tablespoon of coconut oil drops my blood pressure by about 20 points in 30 minutes. I have tested the powerful blood pressure lowering effect of coconut oil on myself numerous times, and it never fails. On one occasion I was rushed to the hospital with dangerously high blood pressure as a result of pain medication. The medicine they injected to lower my blood pressure did not work and they feared I may have a heart attack. I asked to be discharged and went home to take two tablespoons of extra virgin coconut oil. It lowered my blood pressure within half an hour and returned it to normal by the next morning.

As a bonus, I find that the coconut oil gives me more energy at work and I've lost some weight. Please keep me informed of any new developments about coconut oil.

Many thanks,
Efitta Offiong
Ottawa, Ontario

increased energy when the cells receive the nutrients required to function optimally. Another plus is that unrefined virgin coconut oil does not inhibit thyroid function the way unsaturated vegetable oils may. This, again, results in increased energy and also aids in weight management.

The meat from fresh coconut is staple food for islanders of the South Pacific.

Liver

The liver is probably the hardest working of all the body's organs. It detoxifies, secretes hormones, produces bile for digestion of fat, processes vitamins and minerals, and performs literally hundreds more functions vital for maintaining life and proper health. A sluggish liver may result in fatigue, lack of energy, skin disorders, and more.

Unlike other fatty acids, the medium-chain fatty acids in coconut oil are brought straight from the intestines to the liver, bypassing the lymph system where other fats go. The medium-chain fatty acids are burned immediately as fuel and can help liver function in many ways.

The presence of antimicrobial fatty acids, such as those in unrefined virgin coconut oil, can cleanse the liver of harmful microorganisms. High-quality coconut oil will also help to protect the liver from dangerous free radicals.

One study showed that coconut oil can help to prevent alcohol-induced liver damage by inhibiting the formation of free radicals (*Journal of the American College of Nutrition* 2002). Additional research has suggested that coconut oil may also help to rejuvenate damaged liver tissue, including alcohol-related liver damage. Research on animals has shown that medium-chain fatty acids are an effective treatment for hepatitis C infections.

Everyone can enjoy better health by being kind to their liver. Consuming unrefined virgin coconut oil is a delicious way to love your liver and reap the benefits.

Prostate

A great number of men suffer from the effects of an enlarged prostate as they age. Researchers believe that a contributing factor to enlarged prostate in men, or benign prostatic hyperplasia (BPH), involves the hormone dihydrotestosterone (DHT). It

29

appears this male hormone accumulates in the prostate gland and encourages the growth of prostate cells, causing enlargement.

The herb saw palmetto has shown great success in treating enlarged prostate because it blocks the conversion of testosterone into DHT. Since many of the fatty acids found in saw palmetto are medium-chain fatty acids similar to those in coconut, experts believe that coconut oil may work to treat and prevent enlarged prostate as well.

Coconut Oil for Natural Weight Loss

Whenever I talk to people about the many health-promoting and healing benefits of virgin coconut oil, one of the most frequently asked questions is, "Isn't coconut oil a bad saturated fat that's high in calories and will make me fat?" The short answer is no—not if you're consuming high-quality unrefined virgin coconut oil, that is. The reason for this takes a bit of explaining.

What people need to understand is that there's more to weight loss than simple math. The fat-free, low-fat, low-calorie food market, which has failed miserably in terms of helping people to lose weight, is based on such simple thinking. Those who believe that eating less fat will result in fat loss are sadly mistaken. Similarly, counting calories is not the answer. These are not the best measures for weight reduction—biochemistry and metabolism are.

Yes, fat has about twice as many calories per gram as protein or carbohydrates, but there's a lot more to weight gain and weight loss than calories. Fat, along with complex carbohydrates such as the vegetables and grains that supply fibre and nutrients, provides a feeling of satisfaction and helps to reduce cravings for processed carbohydrates. The typical Western diet, high in processed carbohydrates such as soft drinks, refined sugar, and white flour, has led to the astronomical rise in obesity in the entire civilized world. If we are hungry and reach for more carbohydrates than the body can use up for energy, the extra are stored in the body as fat.

A clinical study published in the *American Journal of Clinical Nutrition* (September 2007) showed that eating twice as much fat led to greater weight loss. Researchers compared two eating plans that were similar in caloric intake, but vastly different in fat consumption. Compared with the high-carbohydrate, low-fat diet, the low-carbohydrate, high-fat diet was associated with significantly greater weight loss. Obese individuals who consumed 61 percent of their energy as fat for eight weeks lost an average of 18 pounds each.

Fat will not make you fat—not if it's unrefined virgin coconut oil. In fact, you have to eat fat to lose fat. It's true! Another factor to explain this is that fat comes in different types. As discussed earlier, unrefined virgin coconut oil contains medium-chain fatty acids. These medium chains are easily digested compared to the longer chains found in butter and other animal fats, for example.

Science proves medium-chain fats help weight loss

An interesting clinical study conducted at Charles University in Prague (*Physiological Research* June 1999) proved that the intake of medium-chain fatty acids did not lead to an increase in body weight, and in fact led to weight loss. As a result, the doctors, scientists, and nutritionist involved in the research recommended a weight reduction regimen of 20 grams of virgin coconut oil for the first few days, increasing to 30 grams a day thereafter. (To give you an idea of the size of this portion, picture three of the commonly served 10-gram, individually wrapped butter portions served in restaurants. These would be equal to 30 grams.)

You must be wondering just how much weight you can lose by consuming unrefined virgin coconut oil. Scientists at McGill University in Montreal reviewed all of the scientific literature on this topic and projected that a person could lose 5.4 to 16.2 kilograms (11 to 35 pounds) in a year simply by including medium-chain, fatty acid-rich, virgin coconut oil in his or her diet. I also strongly suggest rigorously avoiding the long-chain fatty acids found in soy, sunflower, peanut, and canola oils, as well as in beef, to ensure and further this possibility.

How, you may be wondering, does coconut oil actually help people lose weight? There is not just one, but many ways eating unrefined virgin coconut oil results in weight loss. First of all, by including virgin coconut oil in your diet, along with essential fatty acids, you provide nourishment to every cell so that your body can function better. You also help to balance hormones, which results in better body functioning and fat burning. Yet another reason high-quality coconut oil aids in weight loss is that it has fewer calories than other forms of fat. Unrefined virgin coconut oil has 6.5 calories per gram, while other fats have 9 calories per gram. Eating this healthy fat also provides a feeling of satisfaction, keeping you from reaching for more food.

Lastly, an important reason unrefined virgin coconut oil helps in weight loss is because it speeds up metabolism. The McGill scientists' review, published in the *Journal of Nutrition* (2002), examined close to thirty studies and found that diets high in medium-chain fatty acids, such as high-quality coconut oil, increase metabolism and favorably affect body fat and weight.

Skin and hair benefits from coconut oil.

Metabolism is the sum of all the chemical processes the body uses to convert food to the nutrients it needs to function, repair, maintain, and grow. The faster this happens the more fuel, including fat, is burned. Many studies have shown that those of us with high metabolisms burn calories more quickly than those with slower rates of metabolism.

Coconut oil weight loss program

Coconut oil is a safe, delicious, healthy way to lose weight. To jumpstart a weight loss program, include approximately 50 percent or more of your fats from unrefined virgin coconut oil. Try three to four tablespoons a day, taken straight (it tastes delicious, so this will not be a problem!), in salad dressing, or blended in a nutritious drink. This dose is

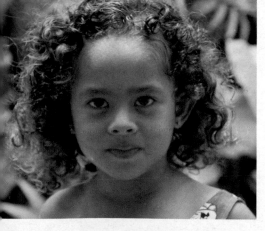

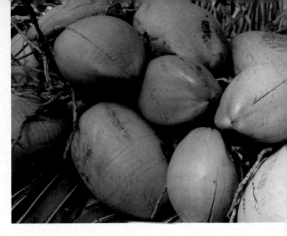

equivalent to eating fresh, shredded coconut meat from half a coconut or drinking a glass of fresh coconut milk. Taking more than the recommended dose makes coconut oil a good detoxifying laxative.

I advise, in addition to the coconut oil weight reduction regime, consuming a diet containing good amounts of fibre from complex carbohydrates (fruit, vegetables, whole grains, and legumes). The majority of saturated fat should come from coconut oil, not animal products. Other dietary fats should contain essential fatty acids, such as those in fresh nuts and seeds and their oils. Including some extra virgin olive oil and freshly pressed flaxseed oil is recommended as well. .

The selection process of fresh mature coconuts ensures the highest quality of virgin oil.

I cannot emphasize enough just how important it is to buy only high-quality fats and oils, no matter what type. Purchase them from merchants you know and trust to provide high quality. Most supermarket brands are rancid and of low quality. These fats are not health promoting, they are cancer causing.

Coconut Oil for Healthy Skin and Hair

I'm always surprised when I'm at health shows to learn how many people know coconut oil as a beauty aid only. They associate it with high-quality cosmetics and as a remedy for improving skin conditions. For these people coconut oil is used topically to ensure soft, radiant skin and lustrous hair.

They are right. Unrefined virgin coconut oil is not just for inner health, but outer health and beauty as well. Coconut oil has been used in the tropics to protect skin from sun and wind for thousands of years. It's no coincidence that tropical people have such beautiful and healthy looking skin and hair.

Traditionally, women in the tropics use unrefined virgin coconut oil not only to keep their skin and hair healthy and beautiful, but also to massage their abdomen during pregnancy. This provides amazing results in the prevention of stretch marks.

When used on the skin, coconut oil absorbs quickly, has a mild, pleasant smell and does not leave the skin feeling greasy or

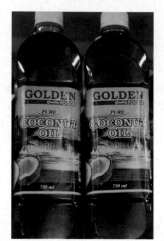

Dark colored coconut oil made from copra does not have the health benefits clear virgin or extra virgin coconut oil has.

34

sticky. Since coconut oil melts easily on the skin, it is a lovely massage oil as well. You can use pure coconut oil for massage, or use it as a base oil and add a small amount of skin-friendly essential oil, such as lavender. Applying a small amount of coconut to the soft skin around the eyes will help to reduce and smooth wrinkles and dry lines.

Whenever East Indian women visit my virgin coconut oil booth at health shows they praise the virtues of this tropical oil for its value in beautifying their hair, for a fraction of the cost of a cupboard full of expensive hair products.

Whether you consider your hair to be your crowning glory, have trouble managing it, or are losing it faster than you'd like, follow the lead of East Indian and Polynesian women and use virgin coconut oil. Apply it to your hair as a pre-shampoo moisturizer and strengthener. Let it sit for a while as you prepare breakfast or take a relaxing bath and then shampoo as normal. Some users prefer to massage coconut oil into their hair and scalp at bedtime and then wash it out with shampoo in the morning.

Some research shows that the medium-chain fatty acid molecules that are plentiful in coconut oil are small enough to easily penetrate hair roots and follicles, adding nourishment and preventing protein loss. Anecdotal evidence clearly shows that coconut oil is also effective in adding softness, luster, and shine as well.

By the way, women who are sold on coconut oil for skin and hair health say men can benefit as well, so don't be shy, guys. Give it a try.

Coconut oil treats skin ailments

Unrefined virgin coconut oil is a miraculous remedy for skin conditions, burns, and injuries. A double-blind study conducted by the Department of Dermatology at the Makati Medical Centre in the Philippines (*Dermatitis* September 2004), concluded that coconut oil is safer and more effective than mineral oil for the treatment of dry skin. The study, which involved 35 patients, also

A village vendor selling copra oil.

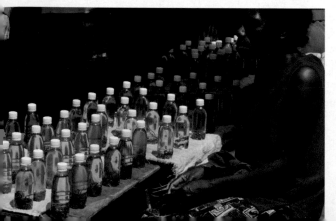

found that coconut oil was the superior choice for rough, scaly, and itchy skin. Coconut oil is a good choice for eczema and even diaper rash.

Dr. Marieta Jader-Onate, founder and CEO of the Good Shepherd Hospital in Lucena City, Philippines, has done a number of clinical trials using coconut oil with patients who have skin conditions. He reports successful treatment of burns, freckles, unidentified brown spots, and psoriasis through antibacterial coconut bath soaps for several months. As a reminder, the lauric acid in coconut oil is antibacterial, antiviral, anti-inflammatory, and also anti-allergenic. Due to these properties, coconut oil is extremely effective on most types of rashes, including diaper rashes.

I have a personal success story when it comes to coconut oil and skin health. After suffering with dry, rough skin on my feet for longer than I'd like to remember, unrefined virgin coconut oil provided fantastic, and fast, relief. Previously, my pain would get so bad that I had trouble walking. Split skin would result in raw wounds. Today, regular massage with coconut oil prevents the nuisance and pain of this condition. With regular attention, athlete's foot, nail infections, and the like can be nipped in the bud.

Use coconut oil as first aid for cuts and abrasions. Simply clean the affected area, thoroughly apply virgin coconut oil, and cover with a coconut oil-saturated bandage. This remedy will allow remarkably quick healing. Coconut oil can also provide quick relief for insect bites and stings.

Ultimately, coconut oil will have the best effect on your skin from the inside out, by using it internally as well as externally. Internal protection means less of the free radical damage that ages skin and contributes to wrinkles.

Quality Counts in Coconut Oil

How can you tell if coconut oil is of high quality or not? It's not easy without some understanding of the production process and some 'clues about the labels. Determining quality is extremely important, however, and means the difference between buying a coconut oil that will help you reach your health goals and one that hinders your efforts.

Reading coconut oil labels can be a confusing and frustrating affair. To date, no official organization, government, or international council exists to grade or standardize the quality of coconut oil, as is the case for olive oil, for instance. However, the Philippine Coconut Authority (PCA) has an official grade distinction outline, which is accepted by other groups, including the Asian and Pacific Coconut Community (APCC). They recognize the differences between low-quality refined, bleached, and deodorized (RBD) coconut oil made from copra, and higher quality virgin coconut oil (VCO).

Dry and dirty

When coconut meat is dried, it's called copra. The coconut meat is dried by smoke, the sun, or in kilns, or a combination of these processes. These processes are not sanitary, which means that when coconut oil is extracted from copra it must be purified (refined). The copra-derived coconut oil is typically filtered to remove impurities, bleached to make it white again (originally it is brown or yellow), and deodorized to eliminate a musty smell. All this is done using high heat. Other dangers include the moulds that may contaminate the copra while it is being shipped to the refining production plants.

The end result is a refined, bleached, and deodorized product, which is why it's known as RBD. This process damages the coconut oil and, to make matters worse, sodium hydroxide (lye) is generally used to prolong shelf life. This, unfortunately, is how 90 percent of all coconut oil on the market today is produced. No wonder health experts and nutritionists who are educated about coconut oil consider refined coconut oil a dead food and recommend unrefined virgin coconut oil.

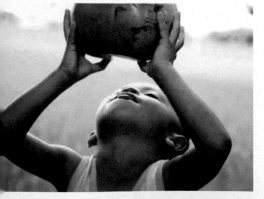

The nutritional value of fresh thirst-quenching coconut water surpasses any manufactured soft drink.

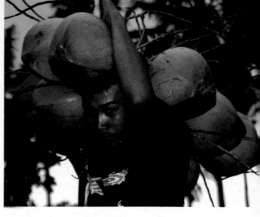

Fresh is best

Prior to 1998 all mass-market coconut oil was produced from copra. Since then, however, there is a much higher quality option being made from fresh, not dried, coconut. This higher quality coconut oil is termed "virgin." Unfortunately, only 10 percent of edible food grade coconut oil is made from fresh coconuts.

The best quality oil is processed from fresh, not dried, coconut.

Virgin coconut oil is extracted directly from the fresh coconut kernel, the fruit of the coconut palm, using some mechanical or other physical means that does not alter the oil.

The Philippine National Standard defines "virgin" coconut oil as being produced:

- from the fresh, mature kernel of the coconut
- by mechanical or natural means
- with or without the use of heat
- without undergoing chemical refining, bleaching or deodorizing, and
- without alteration of the nature of the oil.

Production affects quality

Even though a coconut oil jar says "virgin" and is better than the oil made from copra, there is still a wide range in quality. That's why you see labels that say "virgin," "premium virgin," or "extra virgin."

Most virgin coconut oil is mass-produced from fresh coconut meat by means of expeller pressing. Differences in quality result from whether the nuts are hand selected for ripeness, and from quality control in the manufacturing process. Mass-produced virgin coconut oil involves transporting coconuts from farms to large urban oil mills.

There are two ways of making expeller pressed coconut oil—fresh dry processing and wet milling. To obtain pure oil from coconuts, the water and fat need to be separated. This can be done in very simple operations suitable for village level production or in more sophisticated large-scale manufacturing processes with high capital investments. In the fresh dry process, grated coconuts are dried with air or heat to evaporate the moisture before expeller pressing. In the wet milling method, fresh coconut meat is expeller-pressed first and then further processed, either by heating until the water evaporates, or fermenting until the water separates from the fat. The oil can still be called virgin even if it's filtered and heated. Such processing will, however, affect taste, smell, and quality.

Fermentation is the more traditional method for making virgin coconut oil. As mentioned above, fresh coconuts are pressed to extract coconut milk. The milk is fermented for 24 to 36 hours, until the oil separates from the water and solid matter. The oil is then warmed up to remove any remaining moisture, which will prevent rancidity. The result is natural, unrefined, chemical-free oil. Because this process takes place in open vats, oxygen can affect the flavor, giving some batches a soapy taste.

A jar of coconut oil labeled "premium virgin" indicates a product that is higher quality than virgin, but not as high as extra virgin. Fresh, mature nuts (12 to 13 months old) are used and the oil is produced in factories under strict quality control. The oil has a very nice texture, is pure white, and boasts a beautiful, mild coconut flavour.

Extra virgin coconut oil provides extra quality—and extra health benefits. This high-quality coconut oil is raw oil, produced by either centrifugation or a trademarked process known as direct micro expelling (DME). To my knowledge neither of these processes is currently used in the Philippines. Both of these natural processes require 18 to 20 nuts to produce 1 litre of oil (just over a quart), while the expeller pressing mass-producing method yields 1 litre of oil from only 10 to 12 nuts.

Only DME or centrifuged coconut oil should truly be defined and labeled "extra virgin," because the oil is made from the first, and only, pressing of organically grown coconuts.

In the centrifuge process, fresh coconut meat is grated and pressed to produce coconut milk, which is then placed in a machine that rapidly spins the material to separate the water, solid

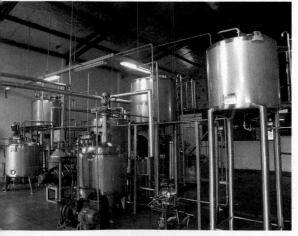

The modern process of centrifuging coconut oil requires sophisticated and expensive equipment.

Cheap Coconut Oil

Sadly, many consumers do not question the detrimental mass production methods that result in low prices (and low quality!). Ideally, people would see that paying more for a higher quality product is immediate health insurance. We all need to recognize that mass produced, heat-treated fats are significant contributors to the degenerative diseases that plague the Western civilized world. Most of us need an immediate oil change! But that's not happening because most people do not shop with their health in mind. Instead, they purchase food according to convenience, flashy packaging, and price. Fortunately, most health food stores offer virgin or extra virgin coconut oil that is often produced with fair trade standards, instead of being mass-produced in oil mills.

material, and oil. The water is then vacuum evaporated. The equipment used for this process has only been perfected in the last two years. The centrifuge process is done under a medium scale plant operation using specially trained operators; therefore, the investment cost for the sophisticated equipment is high. As a result the price for the oil is high, but worth it—it has a very light texture and retains all of its flavour, scent, and health-promoting properties.

The DME process uses a manually operated cold-pressing unit to produce raw oil from fresh coconuts in as little as 90 minutes, or less. Such a short processing time eliminates the concern of mould growth or danger of other impurities. There is no need to refine the oil because it is made on site, where the coconuts grow. No heating, chemical treating, or deodorizing is required. This highest of quality oils boasts a fresh coconut smell and flavour, and retains all of the nutrients required for optimal health. It can be used effectively as a supplement, treatment, or food.

The DME process concentrates on small, manageable daily batches, instead of mass quantities. Such a process depends upon simple, easily learned skills, providing meaningful employment to small teams of people, including families who enjoy working together.

The process is called "direct micro expelling" for the following reasons:

- Direct—Coconut oil is processed directly from fresh coconuts in a quick and efficient process.
- Micro—Small scale, family farms are involved and community members are employed.
- Expelling—Extra virgin oil is extracted by cold pressing.

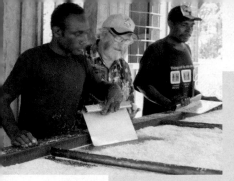

The author watching the drying of freshly grated coconut in preparation for oil pressing.

Unique Production Employs Island Communities

During my extensive research into coconut oil several years ago, I heard the very interesting and inspiring story about DME coconut oil production.

The inventor of the process and the press (called SAM) is Dr. Dan Etherington, an agricultural economist at the Australian National University in Canberra. His interest in eliminating poverty from rural communities and developing healthy oil in an economical way resulted in the DME system. Etherington retired from his teaching post, where he studied and taught the subject of tropical oils, founded the company Kokonut Pacific, and now teaches indigenous people to produce unrefined virgin coconut oil for a living. Successful users of DME technology include coconut farmers on islands in the South Pacific, such as Fiji, Samoa, Tonga, and the Solomon Islands, as well as Indonesia, Kenya, and Sri Lanka.

DME promotes fair trade

It's no wonder Dr. Etherington chose "empowering and bringing hope" as Kokonut Pacific's motto. With the DME system, he ensures that both tropical farm workers and coconut oil consumers significantly benefit from the production of this oil—in quality, fair trade, and, of course, health.

When Dr. Etherington exhibited his system and patented press at the Hanover World Expo 2000, he was awarded a special prize to recognize his Ecologically Sustainable World Project. He empowers native islanders—many of them say that for the first time they have hope for their futures.

The DME system brings coconut oil production back to the farms where the nuts are grown. "The effects are dramatic on the lives of local communities," explains Dr. Etherington. Families are able to work together, using their skills and supporting themselves with a fair wage for making a product they are proud of. "The people on the Solomon Islands, for example, are producing a superb, high-quality oil that is beginning to flow into the international market in significant quantities."

Farmers and producers receive fair returns and the DME process is helping to make poverty in these tropical areas history, while respecting the community and culture of the workers. The system has dramatically increased employment for rural local men, women, and youth, allowing the families to work in their community and better feed and educate their children. This is full and fair trade at its best.

I have personally witnessed how DME technology is implementing fair trade principles for more than ten years now, and how it results in a four- to fivefold increase in the value of coconut exports compared to copra. My wife, Christel, and I visited the Solomon Islands in February 2008 to see firsthand the operation of one of the DME production stations. I was extremely excited to visit such an operation and learn about such a positive development—one that helps those who make the oil and those who consume it. The advent of microprocessing facilities means that for the first time in history coconut farmers in the South Pacific region have an alternative to earning substandard pay for harvesting copra. They are making more than three times the amount they were during their copra wage days.

Loose Labelling

Unfortunately, importers and packagers are not required to reveal their specific manufacturing process, and most will not reveal their production methods when asked. I have discovered that some suppliers use statements, claims, or descriptions that purposely mislead consumers to make their product look as good or better than their competition. Some manufacturers will go so far as to mix low priced refined coconut oil with virgin coconut oil and then label it virgin.

Savvy consumers must compare coconut oil labels. Inquiring about the reputation of the distributor is a good idea, too. After all, your health depends on it. If you find a "virgin" coconut oil that is sold for a price as low as refined coconut oils, leave it on the shelf. Price is a clue to the quality of the contents. The proof, however, is in the taste and the effectiveness of the product. The taste always gives the refined coconut oil producers away. Refined coconut oil has no flavor.

You now understand the different production processes and can distinguish between qualities of expeller pressed, refined, virgin, and extra virgin, but there is other tricky labeling to consider.

"Pure," "100 percent," and "natural"

These labels don't guarantee much in terms of quality. In fact, most commercial grade coconut oils have one or more of these designations on their labels. What is not revealed, in most cases, is that the oil was extracted from copra and has been refined, bleached, and deodorized. One clue is that it has no coconut smell or flavour. I consider copra-extracted oil "dead" and do not recommend it as part of a healthful diet.

"Organic"

If you see the word "organic" on a coconut oil label, note that it only refers to the coconut growing methods, not the oil production process. Some manufacturers take advantage of well meaning, but uninformed consumers by claiming their product is "100 percent organic refined coconut oil." Organic or not, if coconut oil is refined it is damaging to health. In addition to "certified organic," the label should say "extra virgin," "premium virgin," or "virgin."

Coconut Oil in the Kitchen

The distinct coconut flavour you taste when you eat good quality, virgin or extra virgin, raw coconut oil dissipates somewhat when you heat it up for cooking and baking. It does enhance the flavour of your cooked dishes and baked goods, but not in an overpowering way. Gourmet chefs in leading hotels worldwide value this virtue, and they also value the fact that coconut oil is stable enough for high-heat frying.

I spoke earlier about the importance of using high-quality, stable oil for cooking. I must emphasize this point again here. Oils that are high in polyunsaturated fatty acids, such as sesame, sunflower, and safflower oils, even if they are of extremely high quality (which is usually not the case), are dangerous to cook with. These oils are not stable enough to withstand heating. The heat damages the fat, resulting in damaged and dangerous fatty acids.

If you've ever heated up oil and seen smoke coming off your cooking pan, you've witnessed damaged, cancer-causing oil. Coconut oil has a higher smoke point than any other unrefined vegetable oil, at 230 degrees C (446 degrees F). As a comparison, safflower oil smokes at 160 degrees C (374 degrees F), and pumpkinseed and flaxseed oils at 112 degrees C (234 degrees F). Extra

Understanding Organic

There are many organic certifying agencies around the world that have, more or less, set their own rules as to what is considered organic. In many countries only whole foods from organic farmers are eligible for organic certification, while refined and fractionated foods are excluded. This, unfortunately, is not the case in the US or Canada. We have a large variety of processed foods that contain both whole and refined organic ingredients in the same package, with no consideration as to what the food manufacturing process does to the organic ingredients. A coconut may be organic, but if its oil goes through a damaging process it is unhealthful, just as with any refined vegetable or seed oil.

Canadian author Ross Hall, PhD, of McMaster University in Hamilton, Ontario, described in detail in his classic book, *Food For Naught: The Decline in Nutrition* (Vintage Books 1974), how the refining and deodorizing process of seed and vegetable oils at 180 degrees C (356 degrees F) creates dangerous trans fats. One would think that refined, bleached, and deodorized coconut oils, as well as other refined oils, are not worthy of organic certification. Yet in North America, many brands of tasteless refined oils, including coconut oil without the distinct coconut flavor, can be found in organic grocery sections and even in health food stores. Make sure that in addition to being certified organic, your coconut oil is virgin or extra virgin to ensure health and safety.

virgin coconut oils, such DME or centrifuged, which are considered raw coconut oils, should not be heated higher than 160°C (320°F).

The lower the smoke point of an oil, the easier it is to damage the fatty acids. Research tells us that eating damaged fats is a major contributing factor to the development of degenerative disease, including cancer and heart disease.

To cook with unrefined virgin coconut oil, simply heat the oil and test with a slice of onion. Dip the onion into the oil. When the oil sizzles it is hot enough for frying. Do not raise the temperature beyond this point. Once again, smoking oil is dangerous oil.

Use coconut oil for stir-frying, in recipes, to coat cookware, and to grease cookie sheets. You can substitute coconut oil for butter, lard, or any other type of oil in cooking and baking. Coconut oil makes delicious cookies and cakes. Use it on popped corn, too!

The recipe section of this book will give you some ideas for how to use unrefined virgin coconut oil, but really, there's no limit. Before we get to your recipes, however, I'd like to introduce you to an exciting new coconut product—coconut flour.

Coconut Flour Power Discovered

Who would have thought that the leftovers from virgin coconut oil production would be the source of an extremely nutritious, high fibre, gluten-free flour? Dina Masa, a food technologist, and Divina Bawalan, a chemical engineer, obviously thought about it. Then, to the benefit of many, they invented a coconut flour manufacturing process.

Masa, who is manager of the Product Development Department of the Philippine Coconut Authority, explains that up until recently the leftover coconut material from the oil production was fed to animals. Those must have been happy and healthy animals!

Now people are excited about coconut flour—and for good reason. Coconut flour is low in carbohydrates, has more fibre than any other flour, is a good source of protein, is gluten-free, and tastes delicious. Those diagnosed with celiac disease, or who have wheat or gluten intolerances, are certainly benefiting from the recent discovery of coconut flour.

Low-carb high-fibre flour

Coconut flour is ideal for those who follow a low-carbohydrate eating plan. It has fewer digestible carbohydrates (glucose) than any other flour, including soy. It even has fewer digestible carbohydrates than most vegetables. Coconut flour's high amount of indigestible carbohydrates (fibre) passes through the digestive system without adding calories to the body.

Coconut flour has the highest percentage of dietary fibre of any flour, at 61 percent. By comparison, whole-wheat flour contains only 13 percent fibre, and soy flour contains just 10 percent fibre.

Food manufacturers could improve the quality of their products by replacing low-quality fillers and bulking agents with coconut flour. It would make an excellent choice for high-fibre food and snacks as well. Coconut flour can be considered a functional food, since a diet high in fibre has been studied and shown to prevent constipation, manage diabetes, and prevent degenerative disease, such as heart disease and cancer.

The fibre content in coconut flour helps to reduce cholesterol in the body and decrease blood pressure, thus reducing risk of heart disease. Studies have also shown that coconut consumption increases the activity of antioxidants that protect the heart and arteries from the free radical damage that causes atherosclerosis.

Many studies have shown a correlation between high-fibre diets and a lowered incidence of colon cancer. In addition, researchers at the University of Lund in Sweden found that fibre in the diet can absorb the toxins that promote cancer. Fibre helps to keep our intestines, including the colon, clean, healthy and functioning, by regulating bowel movements.

Coconut flour fits into a weight-loss program as well, because its high fibre content adds bulk to a meal and provides a feeling of satisfaction. In addition, fibre, for the most part, is not broken down or digested by humans, and therefore provides no calories. According

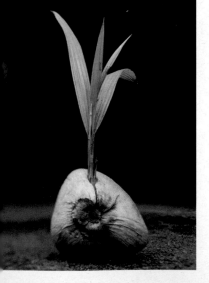

New life sprouts only from a fresh living coconut—equally raw food such as unrefined extra virgin coconut oil promotes good health

44

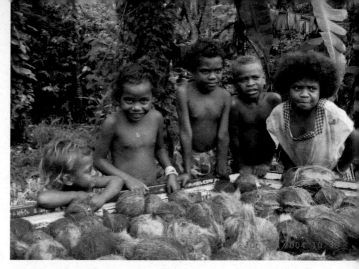

to Dr. Fife, consumption of an additional 14 grams of fibre a day, which is equivalent to ¼ cup of coconut flour, is associated with a 10 percent decrease in calorie intake and a loss in body weight.

Gluten-free flour

The very specific protein known as gluten is found in most grass-related grains, especially wheat, rye, and barley, and including spelt and kamut. Gluten gives dough its elasticity and acts like a kind of glue, helping baked goods to hold together. Gluten also contributes fluffiness to breads, buns, bagels, and muffins.

Children always like to watch where there is excitement.

Although wheat supplies much of the world's dietary protein, a growing percentage of people, including those with celiac disease, are gluten-sensitive or intolerant, which means they cannot properly digest gluten and experience mild to severe reactions as a result. Gluten-free coconut flour is hypoallergenic, safe, and well tolerated by those with celiac disease, sensitivity, intolerance, or even leaky gut syndrome (a condition whereby permeability of the intestinal lining is increased, allowing undigested food particles to enter the bloodstream, and resulting in allergic reaction and health imbalance).

How do you use coconut flour? This gluten-free, high-fibre, low-carb flour can be used to make breads, muffins, cakes, cookies, pies, and other baked goods. Because coconut flour lacks gluten and is highly absorbent it cannot be used as a complete substitute in standard wheat flour recipes. Instead, use coconut flour to replace 15 to 25 percent of other flours in most standard recipes. For breads that require rising, use 10 to 15 percent coconut flour. Coconut flour will help increase the yield of dough because of its high capacity to absorb moisture. I will share some delicious recipes that include coconut flour in the recipe section.

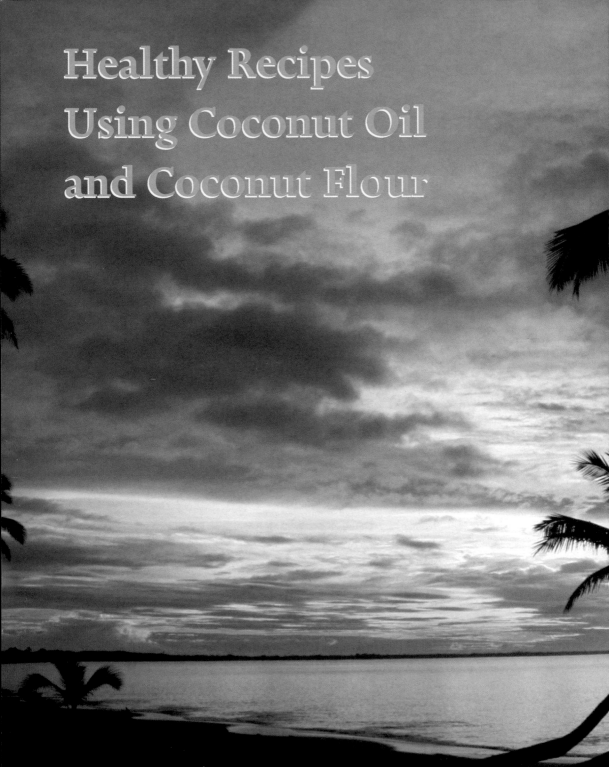

Healthy Recipes
Using Coconut Oil
and Coconut Flour

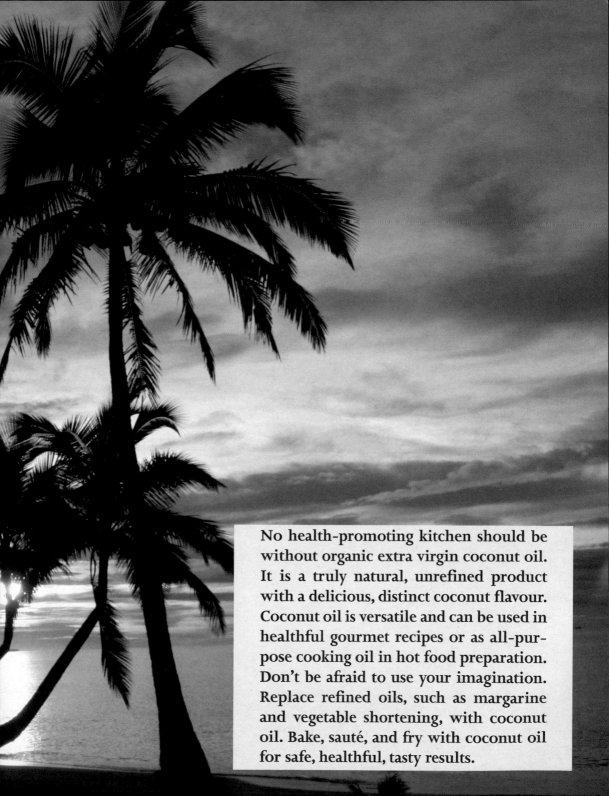

No health-promoting kitchen should be without organic extra virgin coconut oil. It is a truly natural, unrefined product with a delicious, distinct coconut flavour. Coconut oil is versatile and can be used in healthful gourmet recipes or as all-purpose cooking oil in hot food preparation. Don't be afraid to use your imagination. Replace refined oils, such as margarine and vegetable shortening, with coconut oil. Bake, sauté, and fry with coconut oil for safe, healthful, tasty results.

Coconut-Flax Bread Spread

Many people search for a tasty alternative to butter, and I have found this extraordinary option to be exactly that. I especially enjoy it when made with sautéed onions, spread on whole grain bread, and topped with herbal salt. When refrigerated, this spread will stay fresh for several months.

Dr Johanna Budwig, who is famous for her Flax Oil–Protein Diet, used to treat cancer, developed this bread spread. During one of my visits, she impressed on me the nutritional value of the combination of omega-3 fatty acid from flax oil and the short-chain fatty acids of extra virgin coconut oil. She called her coconut–flax oil combination Oleolux. She created the spread to provide her cancer patients with a truly healthy fat that would promote healing and serve as an alternative to dangerous and unhealthy margarine, which is loaded with trans fats. Her own research pointed to trans fats as the culprits in cancer development. Budwig said, "It is the hydrogenation process, creating a molecular change of the naturally occurring cis-form of omega-3 fats in margarine that makes it an unhealthy fat."

As Dr. Budwig handed me her recipe, she emphasized that it is not patented, which meant any company was free to produce and market it. Unfortunately, this bread spread does not lend itself to commercial production, because it easily melts at room temperature. However, it is a tasty alternative to butter and easy to make at home.

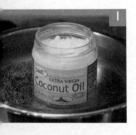

Place the coconut butter in a small container, then set the container in a large bowl of warm water. This will soften the coconut butter and make it easier to work with. Be careful not to let the water run over the sides of the container.

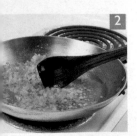

Pour ⅓ of the melted coconut butter into a saucepan over medium heat. Add chopped onion and salt, and sauté, stirring constantly with a wooden spatula until the onions start to brown. Turn the heat down to low and carefully sauté the onions for a few more seconds without letting them burn.

1 cup (250 ml) virgin coconut oil

1 large onion, chopped

1 teaspoon sea salt

½ cup (125 ml) flax oil

10 cloves garlic, minced

Try this spread on fresh rye bread with herbal salt. You'll love it.

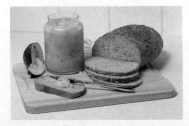

Remove from the heat, let cool to room temperature, and mix with the remaining coconut butter, flax oil and garlic. Pour into a container, seal tightly, and place in the refrigerator. Turn the container upside down every 10 minutes, or stir the spread to prevent the onions from sinking to the bottom.

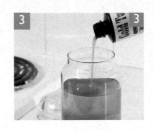

Yield: about 2 cups

Quick Breakfast Bars

A small or quick breakfast doesn't have to be lacking in nutrition. Skip the drive-through window by preparing these quick breakfast bars before a busy week. They are wonderful to wake up to.

1½ cups finely chopped hazelnuts or almonds

1 cup raisins or chopped dried apricots

⅓ cup coconut flour

⅓ cup sesame seeds

¼ cup shredded coconut

1 teaspoon cinnamon

¼ cup organic butter

¼ cup extra virgin coconut oil

¼ cup unpasteurized honey

1 teaspoon vanilla extract

Preheat the oven to 175 degrees C (350 degrees F). Grease an 8-inch square baking dish with coconut oil. Combine the nuts, raisins, flour, sesame seeds, shredded coconut, and cinnamon in a medium bowl. Melt the butter, coconut oil, and honey in a small saucepan over medium heat, and mix well. Add the vanilla and stir. Pour the liquid ingredients over the flour and nut mixture, and mix well. Press the mixture into the prepared dish. Bake for 20 to 25 minutes or until set. Allow to cool before cutting into bars.

Yield: 8 (2 x 4-inch) bars

Breakfast Crème or Smoothie for Two

This is a very satisfying breakfast, combining a good ratio of healthful carbohydrates, protein, and fats. You may eat this delicious crème in bowls or, if you prefer to drink your breakfast, simply add more juice and serve as a smoothie.

½ cup hazelnuts

1 apple, unpeeled, cut into chunks

½ banana

⅔ cup (165 ml) celery, cut in ½" (1 cm) chunks

1 cup fruit juice

3 to 4 tablespoons extra virgin coconut oil (solid)

½ cup cottage cheese, quark, or kefir

Fresh fruit or berries for topping (optional)

Place the hazelnuts in a blender and chop, then add the apple, banana, half of the juice, the cottage cheese, and coconut oil. Blend until smooth. Check the consistency and add the remaining juice, if desired. Pour into small bowls and top with fruit or berries (if using).

Yield: 2 servings

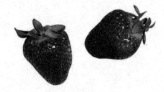

Quark is a soft, fresh fermented cheese that originated in Central Europe. Kefir is a fermented milk drink. Both contain beneficial bacteria that are good for digestion.

To make quark at home, simply pour one or two litres (quarts) of buttermilk or naturally soured milk into a glass jar. Place the jar in a warm oven at a low temperature (about 65 degrees C/150 degrees F) for about eight hours, until the milk solids have separated from the whey. Remove from the oven, let cool off, and ladle the milk solids into a very fine strainer or cheese cloth. Let strain for 24 hours and refrigerate—you will have the spreadable soft cheese called quark.

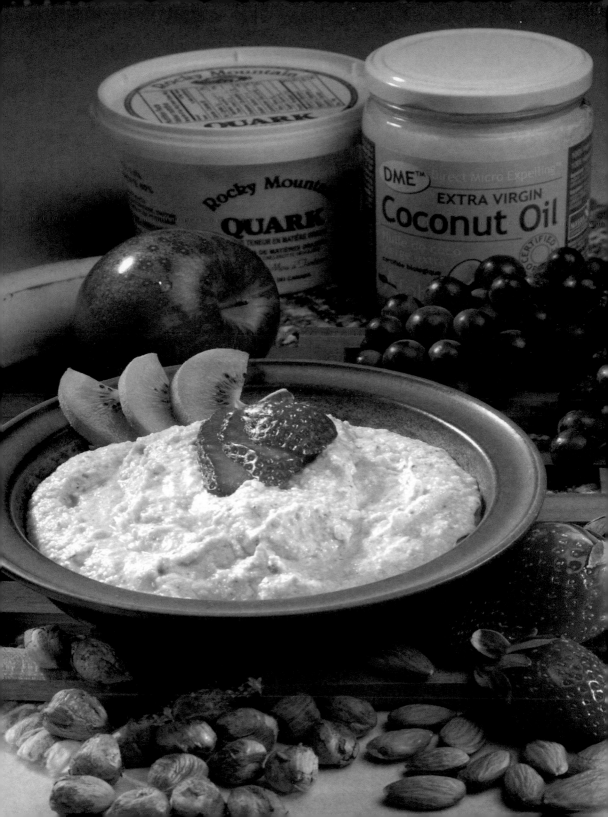

Tropical Breakfast Smoothie

Nothing beats a sit-down, complete nutritious breakfast that includes fresh fruit and fresh, natural cereal. However, for those days when you're on the go, a breakfast smoothie is the next best thing.

1 banana or ½ cup seasonal fruit (blueberries, peaches, etc.)

2 to 3 tablespoons extra virgin coconut oil (solid or liquid)

8 ounces fresh fruit juice

1 teaspoon fibre powder

1 scoop protein powder

Place all the ingredients in a blender and process until smooth.

Yield: 1 serving

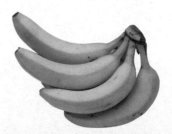

For a less sweet smoothie, substitute 4 ounces juice and 4 ounces water or 8 ounces of rice milk for the juice.

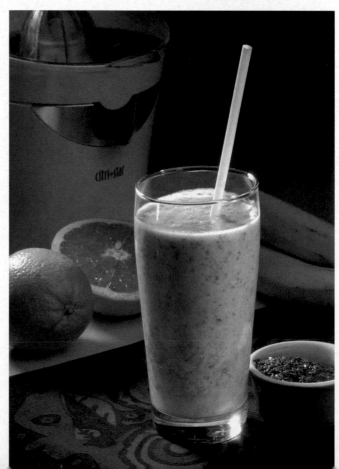

Siegfried's Ranch Salad Dressing

Making your own salad dressing will save you money and save your health. This creamy creation is easy to make and digest, and it's absolutely delicious.

¾ cup extra virgin coconut oil

¼ cup organic, cold-pressed flaxseed oil or hempseed oil

2 eggs

Juice of 1 lemon or 1 lime

2 teaspoons apple cider vinegar or wine vinegar

½ teaspoon Dijon mustard

¼ teaspoon vegetable salt (such as Herbamare or Spike Seasoning)

Dash soy sauce

Combine the coconut oil and flaxseed oil in a small bowl. (If you have to melt the coconut oil first to measure it, simply place the jar in a bowl of hot tap water.) Place the eggs, lemon juice, mustard, salt, and soy sauce in a blender, and process for 10 seconds. With the blender running, slowly add the oil mixture into the blender, and process until smooth. (If the oil is added too fast, the dressing will curdle.) This dressing will keep for 4 to 6 days in the refrigerator.

Yield: 1¼ cups

Coconut Mayonnaise

This unique mayonnaise is both nourishing and satisfying. The secret to making good mayonnaise is to add the oil slowly, which will thicken the mayonnaise.

1 cup extra virgin coconut oil

¼ cup extra-virgin olive oil or hemp oil

2 egg yolks

2 tablespoons lemon juice

½ tablespoon Dijon mustard

⅛ teaspoon paprika

⅛ teaspoon sea salt

This mayonnaise will keep for up to a week, stored in the refrigerator, and will remain soft and spreadable.

Combine the coconut oil and olive oil in a small bowl. (If you have to melt the coconut oil first to measure it, simply place the jar in a bowl of hot tap water.) Place the egg yolks, lemon juice, mustard, paprika, and salt in a blender, and process for 10 seconds. With the blender running, slowly add the oil mixture by pouring a fine, steady stream; this should take 50 seconds.

Yield: 1½ cups

Pacific Rim Rice

Coconut oil and coconut milk add quality fat and taste to this wonderfully tropical pilaf. Serve this to dinner guests and you'll soon be known for this unique dish.

3 tablespoons extra virgin coconut oil

1 onion, finely chopped

1 green bell pepper, finely chopped

¾ teaspoon curry powder

3 cups vegetable broth, hot

1½ cups brown basmati rice

¾ cup unsweetened coconut milk

¼ teaspoon sea salt

1 cup pineapple chunks

¼ cup chopped cashews

Heat the coconut oil in a 3-quart saucepan over medium heat, add the onion and bell pepper, and sauté until the onion is golden brown. Stir in the curry powder and sauté 1 minute. Increase the heat and add the vegetable broth slowly, stirring, until the mixture comes to a simmer. Add the rice, coconut milk, and salt. Lower the heat, cover, and return to a simmer. Cook, without stirring, about 45 minutes, or until all the liquid has been absorbed and the rice is tender. Remove from the heat, stir in the pineapple and cashews, and let sit, covered, for 5 minutes before serving.

Yield: 2 large or 4 small servings

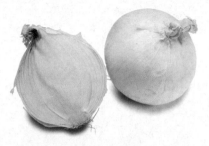

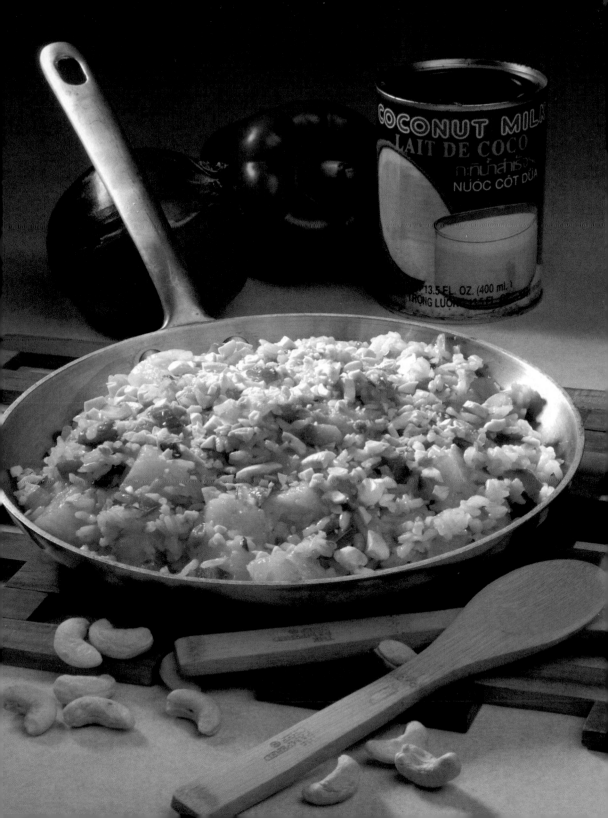

Quinoa and Vegetables

An ancient grain, quinoa originated in South America. It has the highest protein content of all grains and boasts a slightly nutty flavor. Look for it in natural food stores and try this delicious creation, which offers a good amount of beneficial phytonutrients.

1 cup quinoa

¼ cup extra virgin coconut oil

2 cups hot vegetable broth

1 medium onion, coarsely diced

1 green or red bell pepper, diced

1 cup broccoli florets

1 cup sliced mushrooms

Rinse the quinoa thoroughly and drain well. Place the quinoa in a large, heavy skillet over medium heat and toast, stirring continuously, to remove any moisture. Add the coconut oil and sauté the quinoa until it starts to turn golden. Turn off the heat and slowly add the broth. Add the onion, bell pepper, broccoli, and mushrooms, stir, and return the pan to low heat. Cover and simmer for 20 minutes, or until all the moisture has been absorbed.

Yield: 2 large or 4 small servings

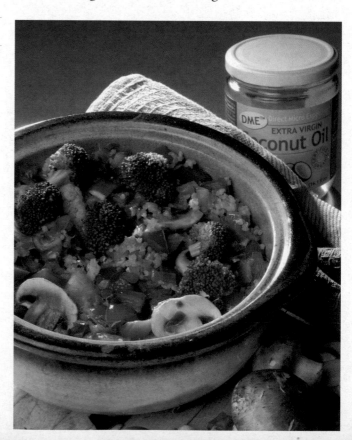

Sesame Coconut Cookies

This gluten-free cookie recipe calls for the use of tahini, which is sesame seed butter. Make sure to buy raw, not roasted, tahini.

1 cup grated or flaked coconut

½ to 1 cup unpasteurized honey (to desired sweetness)

½ cup tahini

½ cup sesame seeds

Dash sea salt

½ cup coconut flour, sifted

Preheat the oven to 175 degrees C (350 degrees F). Grease a cookie sheet with coconut oil and set aside. Place the coconut, the desired amount of honey, the tahini, sesame seeds, and salt in a bowl and stir to blend, then stir in the coconut flour. The batter will be sticky. Drop the batter by spoonfuls on the prepared cookie sheet, 2 inches apart. Bake for approximately 15 minutes or until golden brown. Let the cookies cool before removing them from the cookie sheet.

Yield: about 25 cookies

To give this recipe a more mellow sweetness, replace the honey with ½ cup gluten-free brown rice syrup. If desired, you can use peanut butter or another nut butter in place of the tahini.

Coconut Shortbread Cookies

Coconut oil can easily replace butter in cookie recipes, such as this traditional favourite.

2 cups whole wheat flour

1 cup coconut flour

1 cup premium virgin coconut oil

¼ cup evaporated cane juice (such as Rapadura or Sucanat)

1 teaspoon vanilla extract

½ teaspoon sea salt

¼ teaspoon aluminum-free baking powder

Preheat the oven to 175 degrees C (350 degrees F). Mix all the ingredients together. Pat out into an ungreased 9 x 13-inch baking pan. Bake for 20 to 25 minutes, or until lightly browned. Let cool slightly, then cut into squares and let cool completely.

Yield: 20 to 24 cookies

Double-Crust Apple Pie

Mixing coconut and butter in this pie crust results in a rich, but light, crust taste and texture. This pie tastes great served warm as is, or with a dollop of whipped cream or scoop of ice cream.

Filling

8 medium aromatic apples, such as Braeburn or Macintosh, peeled and cored

1 tablespoon organic butter

1 tablespoon unpasteurized honey or evaporated cane juice (such as Sucanat or Rapadura)

1 teaspoon ground cinnamon

Crust

2 cups whole wheat flour

¾ teaspoon sea salt

⅓ cup coconut oil, cold

⅓ cup butter, cold

5 tablespoons cold filtered water

Yield: one 9-inch pie

To make the filling: Slice each apple into 16 wedges. Heat the butter in a large skillet or pot over medium heat. Add the sliced apples to the skillet and stir to coat with the butter. Cover the pot tightly and cook, stirring gently and frequently for 5 to 7 minutes, until the apples have softened slightly but are still somewhat firm. Add the honey and cinnamon, increase the heat to medium-high, and continue cooking the apples for 3 minutes. Remove from the stove and spread the apples in a thin layer on a baking sheet to cool to room temperature.

To make the crust: Preheat the oven to 205 degrees C (400 degrees F). Grease a 9-inch pie plate with coconut oil. Place the flour and salt in a large bowl, and whisk to blend. Work in the chilled coconut oil and butter with a pastry cutter or fork until the mixture resembles small crumbs, then add the cold water gradually. Knead the dough for 1 minute, then divide in half and form each half into a disk.

Roll out each disk between 2 sheets of waxed paper or parchment paper—one to a 10-inch circle and the other to a 9-inch circle. Place the 10-inch circle into the prepared pie plate. Spoon the apple filling into the pie shell, and cover with the 9-inch circle of dough. Fold the edges of the dough under and seal by pressing with your thumbs or a fork. Cut air vents in the top crust. Bake for 30 to 40 minutes or until the crust is golden brown and the filling is bubbling. Let cool slightly on a wire rack before serving.

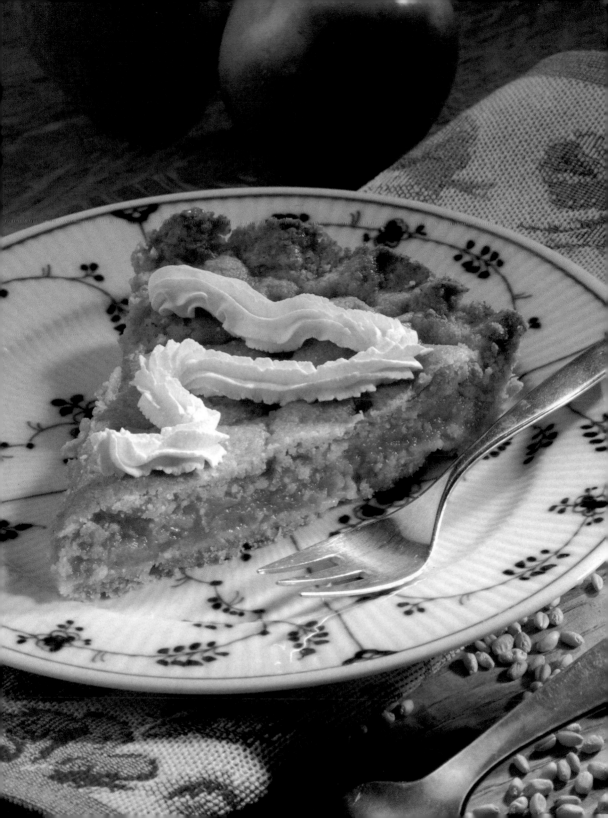

Fruit Sherbet

This cool treat is packed with fibre, phytonutrients and, of course, flavor.

2 bananas, peeled and frozen overnight

1 cup frozen blueberries

8 large frozen strawberries

4 tablespoons extra virgin coconut oil (room temperature)

Whipped cream (optional)

Prepare a twin gear juicer or a single auger juicer for making frozen desserts according to the manufacturer's directions.

Starting with one frozen banana, alternate putting frozen fruit and coconut oil through the juicer. Catch fruit strings in a bowl and place in serving dishes. Serve immediately with a dollop of whipped cream (if using).

Yield: 4 to 6 servings

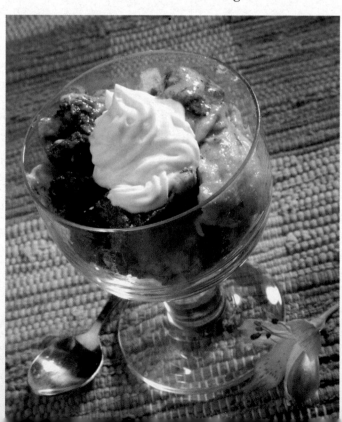

Raspberry Energy Balls

Excellent as snacks or even as a dessert, these tasty coconut-covered balls provide energy and nourishment.

1¼ cup raisins

4 tablespoons dried currants

1 cup sunflower seeds

1 cup pumpkin seeds

½ cup sesame seeds

½ cup raspberries, pureed

3 tablespoons extra virgin coconut oil

3 tablespoons cashew butter

2 tablespoons coconut flour

½ cup finely shredded coconut

Bring 2 cups water to a boil. Place the raisins in a small bowl and add half the water; place the currants in another small bowl and add the remaining water. Let the raisins and currants soak 5 minutes, then drain each separately, reserving the raisin soaking liquid. Process all the seeds in a blender until medium ground. Place the cooled raisins in the blender and add just enough soaking water to process. Scrape the raisin mixture into a medium bowl, add the ground seeds, raspberry puree, coconut oil, cashew butter, coconut flour, and cooled currants, and mix well. Using your hands, roll the mixture into walnut-sized balls (about 1½ inches) and then roll each ball in shredded coconut until completely covered. Freeze; thaw just before serving.

Yield: 32 balls

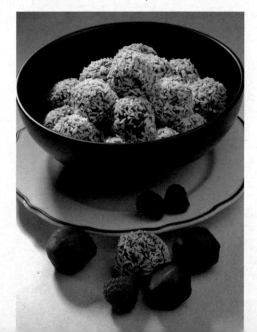

Coconut Energy Bars

Delicious and nutritious, these coconut bars provide fuel and satisfy your sweet tooth, too.

¼ cup extra virgin coconut oil

1½ cups organic semi-sweet chocolate chips

½ cup unpasteurized honey

½ cup almond butter

1¾ cups nuts and/or seeds (pecans, hazelnuts, almonds, sunflower seeds, etc.)

1¼ cups shredded unsweetened coconut

1 cup quick oats

1 teaspoon vanilla extract

Grease a 9 x 13-inch baking pan with coconut oil and set aside. Melt the coconut oil in a medium saucepan over medium-low heat, then stir in the chocolate chips, honey, and almond butter. Bring to a low boil stirring constantly, for 2 to 3 minutes. Remove from the heat and mix in the nuts, coconut, and oats. Turn into the prepared pan. Spread and press firmly. Allow to cool and cut into bars.

Yield: about 20 bars

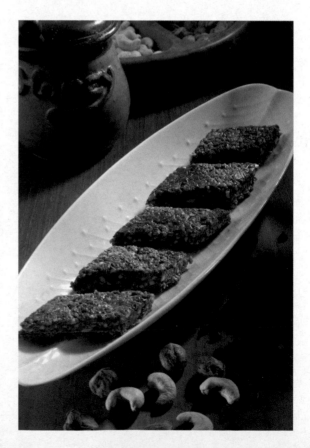

references resources

Agero AL and Verallo-Rowell VM. Department of Dermatology, Makati Medical Center, Makati City, Philippines. *Dermatitis*, 15(3):109-16, September 2004.

Bláha V, et al. *Physiol. Res.* 48: 457-463, June 1999.

Dileep S, Sachan, Ayub M,. Yatim, and Daily JW. *Journal of the American College of Nutrition*. Vol. 21, No. 3, 233-238, 2002.

Halyburton AK, et al. *American Journal of Clinical Nutrition* Vol. 86, No. 3, 580-587, September 2007.

Kabara JJ. *Indian Coconut Journal*, 31(8):2-8, 2000.

Kaunitz H. *Environ Pathol Toxicol Oncol*. 1986 Mar-Apr;6(3-4):115-21..

Lichtenstein AH and Van Horn L. *Circulation*. 1998,98(9):935-9.

Nelson SE, Rogers RR, Frantz JA and Ziegler EE. *American Journal of Clinical Nutrition*. Vol 64, 291-296, September 1996.

Ogbolu, DO, et. al. *Journal of Medicinal Food*. Volume 10: 384-387, No. 2, June, 2007.

Padmakumaran KG, Nair, Rajamohan T, and Kurup PA. *Plant Foods for Human Nutrition*, Volume 53, Number 2 / June 1998.

Polak J, et al. *Journal of Lipid Research*, Vol. 48, 2236-2246, October 2007.

Sadeghi S, et al. *Immunology*, 96(3):404-10, March 1999.

Sales TR, Torres HO, Couto CM, Carvalho EB. *Nutrition*, 14(6):508-12. June 1998..

Sircar S, Kansra U, Department of Medicine, Safdarjang Hospital, New Delhi. *Journal of the Indian Medical Association*. 96(10):304-7. October, 1998.

St-Onge MP and Jones PJH. The American Society for Nutritional Sciences. *The Journal of Nutrition*, 132:329-332, 2002.

Coconut Oil, Coconut Flour, and Related Products

Alpha Health Products Ltd

7434 Fraser Park Drive
Burnaby, BC V5J 5B9
CANADA
Tel: 604-436-0545
or 800-663-2212
Fax: 604-435-4862
E-mail: info@alphahealth.ca
www.alphahealthproducts.ca
or www.cocnutoilandhealth.com

Kokonut Pacific Pty Ltd

PO Box 4088
Hawker, ACT 2614
AUSTRALIA
Tel: +61 2 6254 5606
Fax: +61 2 6255 2651
E-mail:
richard@kokonutpacific.com.au
www.kokonutpacific.com.au

C.W. Tropicai GmbH

Schlesier Str. 5
86637 Wertingen,
GERMANY
Tel: +49-(0)8272-992026
Fax:+49-(0)8272-992306
E-mail: info@tropicai.com
Web site: www.tropicai.com

South Pacific Trading

15052 Ronnie Drive #100
Dade City, FL 33523
USA
Tel: 352-567-2200
www.simplycoconut.com

Tribest Corporation

1143 North Patt Street
Anaheim, CA 92801
USA
Tel: 714.879.7150
Fax: 714.879.7140
E-mail: jae@tribest.com
www.tribest.com

For all other coconut inquiries

The Coconut Research Center

P.O. Box 25203
Colorado Springs CO 80936
USA
Tel: 719-550-9887
www.coconutresearchcenter.org

Published by **Books Alive**
PO Box 99
Summertown, TN 38483
(931) 964-3571
(888) 260-8458

Book Design/Artwork:
    Cord Slatton
    Warren Jefferson
Art Direction:
    Siegfried Gursche
Recipe Development:
    Siegfried Gursche
    Christel Gursche
    Pat Roman
Food Preparation:
    Christel Gursche
Food Styling:
    Emond Fong
    Christel Gursche
Photography:
    Edmond Fong (recipe)
    Siegfried Gursche (editorial)
    Warren Jefferson (cover)
    Dr. Renato M. Labadan
Photo Editing:
    Cord Slatton
Editing:
    Sandra Tonn
    Cheryl Redmond

Library of Congress Cataloging-in-Publication Data

Gursche, Siegfried, 1933-
  Coconut oil : discover the key to vibrant health / Siegfried Gursche.
      p. cm. -- (Alive natural health guides ; 37)
  ISBN 978-1-55312-043-8
  1. Coconut oil--Health aspects. 2. Fatty acids in human nutrition. 3. Cookery (Coconut oil) I. Title.

  QP144.O44G86 2008
  612.3'97--dc22   2008015495

Printed in Hong Kong

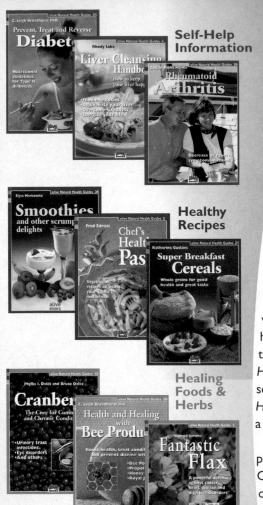

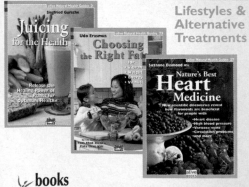

alive Natural Health Guides

Self-Help Information

Healthy Recipes

Healing Foods & Herbs

Lifestyles & Alternative Treatments

About this author ....

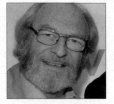

Long acknowledged as the father of the Canadian health food movement, Siegfried Gursche comes by his vast amount of knowledge about healthy fats and oils through both firsthand experience and dedicated research. Gursche founded the original *alive* Canadian Journal of Health and Nutrition, *alive* Books, and *alive* Academy of Nutrition—all of which helped so many take health into their own hands. He researched, commissioned, and published the world-renowned book by Udo Erasmus, *Fats that Heal, Fats that Kill*, the *alive* Natural Health Guides series, and the award-winning *Encyclopedia of Natural Healing*, all of which are now published by Books Alive, a division of Book Publishing Company.

In addition to his writing efforts to educate people about natural health and nutrition, Gursche is the Canadian distributor, through Alpha Health Products, of high-quality organic fair trade DME Extra Virgin Coconut Oil. He practices what he teaches and is happy to share his knowledge in this practical, easy-to-understand, and up-to-date guide on this important topic.

About this series ....

The ***Alive Natural Health Guides*** is the first series of its kind in North America. Each book focuses on a specific natural health related topic and explains how you can improve your health and lifestyle through diet and natural healing methods.

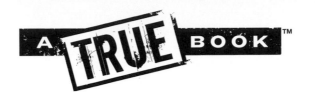

A TRUE BOOK™

The Confederate States of America

PETER BENOIT

Children's Press®
An Imprint of Scholastic Inc.
New York Toronto London Auckland Sydney
Mexico City New Delhi Hong Kong
Danbury, Connecticut

Content Consultant
James Marten, PhD
Professor and Chair, History Department
Marquette University
Milwaukee, Wisconsin

Library of Congress Cataloging-in-Publication Data

Benoit, Peter, 1955–
   The Confederate States of America/Peter Benoit.
      p. cm. — (A true book)
   Includes bibliographical references and index.
   ISBN-13: 978-0-531-26310-5 (lib. bdg.)   ISBN-10: 0-531-26310-X (lib. bdg.)
   ISBN-10: 978-0-531-26623-6 (pbk.)   ISBN-10: 0-531-26623-0 (pbk.)
   1. Confederate States of America—History—Juvenile literature. 2. United States—History—Civil
War, 1861–1865—Juvenile literature. I. Title.
   E487.B46 2012
   973.7'13—dc22   2011011968

Find the Truth!

Everything you are about to read is true *except* for one of the sentences on this page.

Which one is **TRUE**?

T or F   The Confederate States of America were formed before President Abraham Lincoln took office.

T or F   Confederate president Jefferson Davis was executed after the Civil War.

Find the answers in this book.

3

Contents

THE **BIG** TRUTH!

Slavery in the South

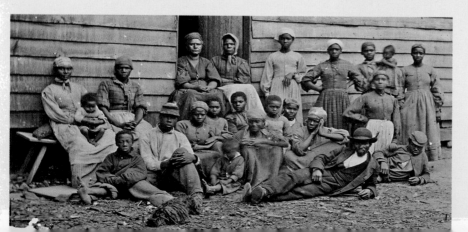

**Enslaved
African
Americans**

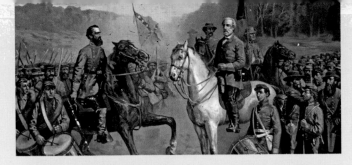

Confederate generals

3 The Confederate Government

4 The End of an Era

The Confederate States of America issued its first currency in April 1861.

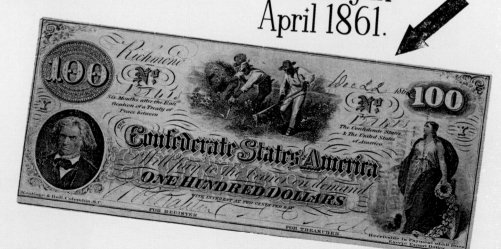

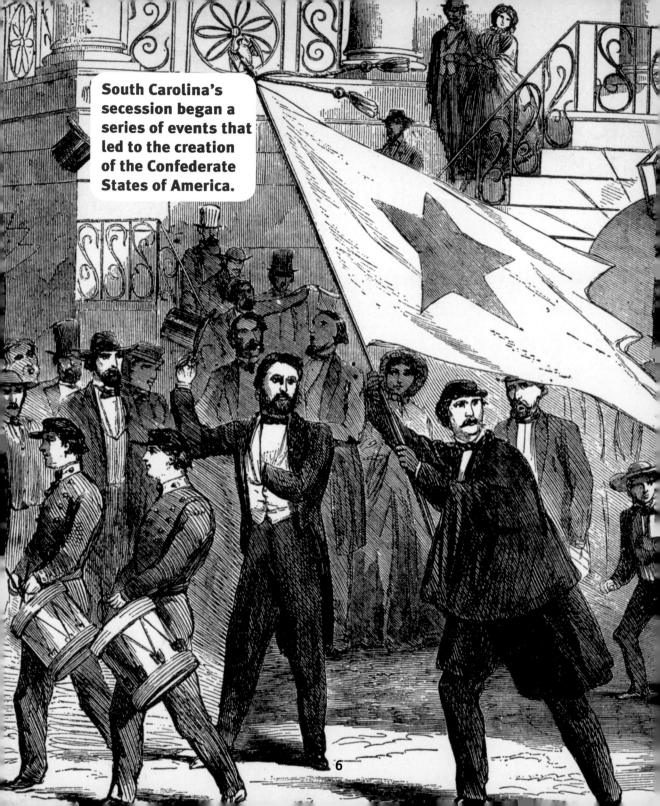

South Carolina's secession began a series of events that led to the creation of the Confederate States of America.

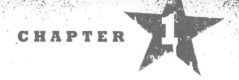

Seeds of Secession

The state of South Carolina **seceded** from the United States of America on December 20, 1860. This set off a chain of events that led to 11 states leaving the Union to form a new nation called the Confederate States of America. South Carolina's decision to leave the Union was not made suddenly. It happened after years of disagreement between the northern and southern states about how the country should be run.

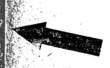

Secessionists created new flags to show support for states' rights.

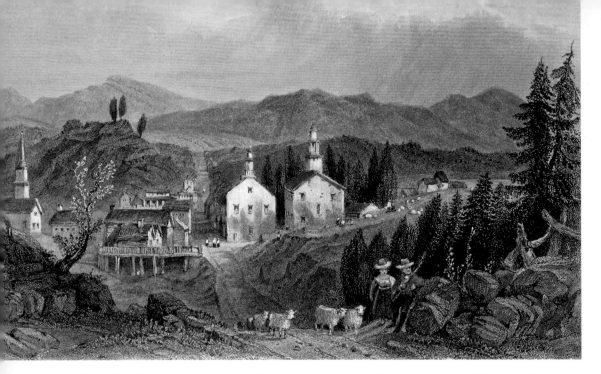

Rural villages were much more common than larger cities and towns in the early years of the United States.

States' Rights

Americans had disagreed for years over which powers should belong to the states and which should belong to the **federal** government. These differences did not cause major problems at first. Most of the country's settlements consisted of farms and small villages. People from different states did not often communicate with one another.

This lack of communication led to the states creating their own rules and developing in their own ways. Each state passed laws that suited its people and **economy**. The federal government did not often take part in this process. Most southern states' economies were based on agriculture. Some farms were small. But others were large **plantations**. They produced crops such as cotton, sugar, and tobacco.

Before the Civil War, Louisiana produced between 25 and 50 percent of all sugar used in the United States.

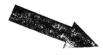

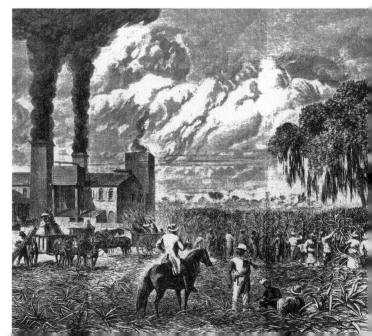

Trade and Slavery

The economy in the South depended on two things to make it work. The first was trade with foreign countries. Great Britain purchased huge amounts of cotton and tobacco from the southern states. The second was slavery. Slavery was important because southern farmers and plantation owners relied on slaves to produce their crops. Slavery was not allowed in most of the northern states. But millions of slaves were forced to work on southern farms.

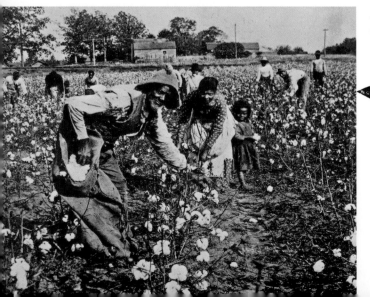

Slaves were forced to do difficult, tiring jobs such as picking cotton.

The U.S. slave population was more than four million by the beginning of the Civil War.

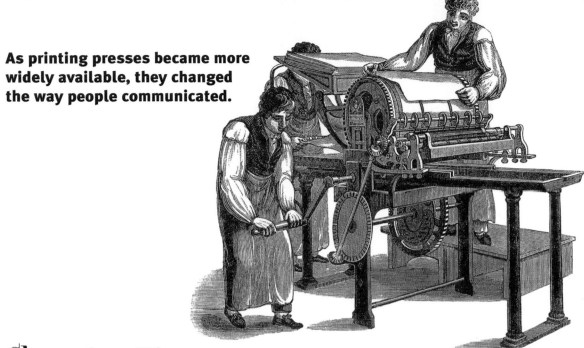

As printing presses became more widely available, they changed the way people communicated.

Changing Times

Advances in communication and transportation began to have major effects on the country in the early 1800s. Railroads and the printing press made it easy for people to learn what was happening across the country. People began to develop opinions about the other states' ways of doing things. The federal government eventually started to take a more active role in the country's lawmaking process.

Tariff Trouble

The U.S. government created a new **tariff** on imported goods in 1828. It had previously been cheaper to import goods from foreign countries than to get the same goods from the manufacturers in the northern United States. The tariff was designed to protect these U.S. companies from going out of business. The results of the tariff eventually harmed the southern agricultural economy.

Tariffs were designed to help U.S. manufacturing businesses by making foreign-manufactured goods more expensive.

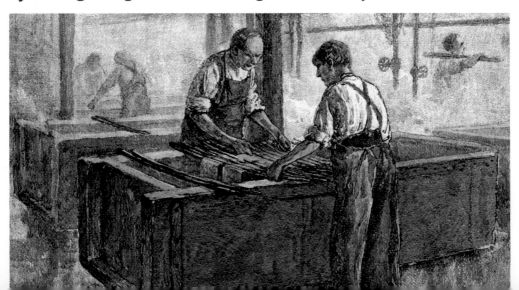

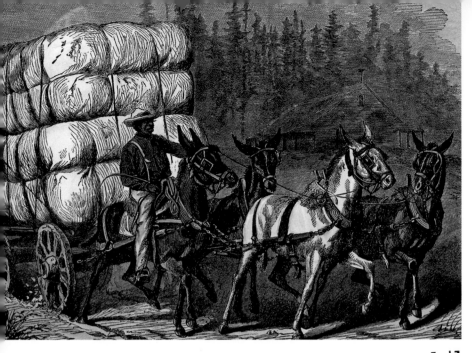

The tariffs made it hard for plantation owners to sell their crops.

Many southerners called the tariff "The Tariff of Abominations."

People in the southern states were now forced to purchase more expensive goods from the north. Manufacturers in countries such as Great Britain began to lose money as Americans purchased fewer of their products. This left foreign nations with less money to buy crops from the southern states. The southerners feared that this would hurt their economy as time went on.

The Nullification Crisis

Protests from the south led to the U.S. government lowering the tariff in 1832. But this did not satisfy all southerners. The South Carolina state government passed the Ordinance of **Nullification**. It stated that the tariffs would not apply in that state. It also threatened that the

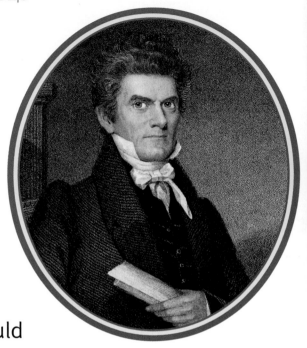

U.S. vice president John C. Calhoun spoke out in favor of nullification.

state would secede if the U.S. government tried to force them to pay the tariff. No other states joined South Carolina in this protest. State leaders were pressured into canceling it.

Regional Tensions

South Carolina's actions showed that there was a large difference between northern and southern states. The issue of slavery divided the North and South even further over the next 25 years. New territories were added to the western part of the country. There was debate on whether or not to allow slavery in those locations. Many people in the north were against slavery. The South believed that the North was attacking its slave-based economy.

After the Civil War, Senator Sumner supported the right for former slaves to vote.

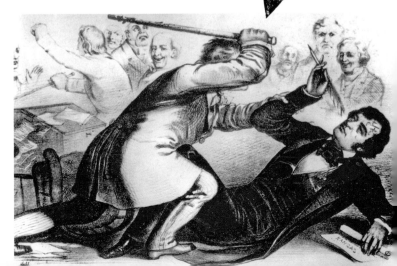

In 1856, South Carolina congressman Preston S. Brooks attacked Massachusetts senator Charles Sumner with a cane over a disagreement about states' rights.

CHAPTER 2

The Birth of the Confederate States of America

The Confederate States of America was often called simply the Confederacy. It was born out of the southern fear of **abolition**. Abolitionists hoped to do away with slavery completely. Abolitionists and southern slaveholders had totally different beliefs. William Lloyd Garrison was the editor of an abolitionist newspaper called the *Liberator*. Garrison wrote that he was filled with "indignation

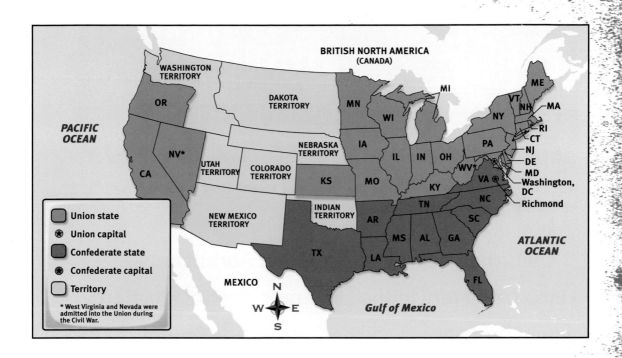

This map shows the Union and Confederate states during the Civil War (1861–1865).

and abhorrence" at "that which turns a man into a thing." But U.S. representative Alexander Stephens of Georgia described slavery as a "natural and normal condition."

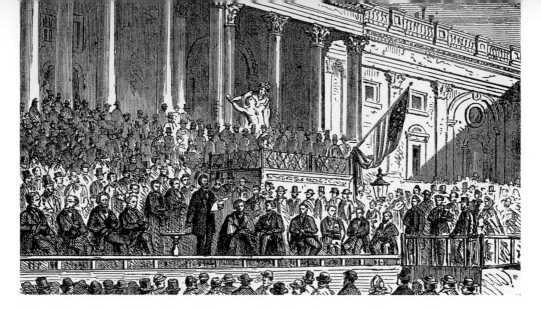

Abraham Lincoln's election was the final event that made some southern states secede from the Union.

Southern leaders feared that Abraham Lincoln's victory in the 1860 presidential election would bring about the end of slavery. Southern slaveholders had previously had a controlling influence in the Supreme Court. They also had powerful backing in Congress. The South believed Lincoln's election would put control in the hands of those who were against slavery. Some states believed secession was the only way to preserve slavery against the threat of the abolitionists.

Support for secession was divided. Extremists such as Alabama congressman William Lowndes Yancey threatened secession if Lincoln won the election. Such extremists were known as Fire-Eaters. Other groups took a more moderate position. They wished to avoid secession until all slave states agreed. A mixture of Union supporters and secessionists helped prevent secession plans in some border states.

Yancey later served as a Confederate diplomat to Europe during the Civil War.

William Lowndes Yancey was one of the most public supporters of secession.

South Carolina led the way toward secession. It started by denying the power of federal judges in their state. Then its two U.S. senators quit. South Carolina seceded from the Union on December 20, 1860. Mississippi, Florida, Alabama, Georgia, Louisiana, and Texas had

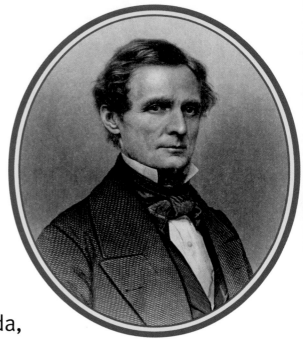

Jefferson Davis was the first and only president of the Confederacy.

all followed by February 1861. **Delegates** from the seven states formed the Confederate States of America. Former Mississippi senator Jefferson Davis was named president of the Confederacy.

The Cornerstone Speech

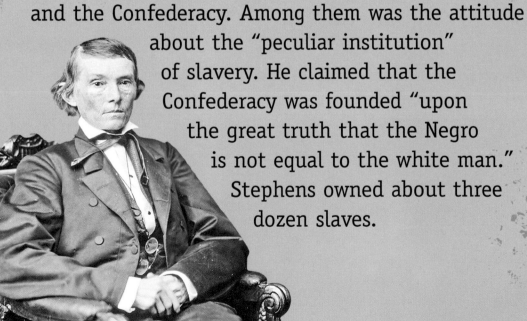

On March 21, 1861, Confederate vice president Alexander Stephens delivered his famous Cornerstone Speech in Savannah, Georgia. He spoke about differences between the U.S. federal government and the Confederacy. Among them was the attitude about the "peculiar institution" of slavery. He claimed that the Confederacy was founded "upon the great truth that the Negro is not equal to the white man." Stephens owned about three dozen slaves.

Lincoln took office on March 4, 1861. U.S. troops at Fort Sumter in Charleston, South Carolina, requested supplies shortly afterward. Fort Sumter was one of the few remaining Union military bases on Confederate soil. Lincoln notified South Carolina governor Francis Pickens of the operation. But Pickens suspected that Lincoln would try to send weapons and troops. The Confederates attacked the fort on April 12.

The attack on Fort Sumter marked the beginning of the Civil War.

No one died during the attack on Fort Sumter.

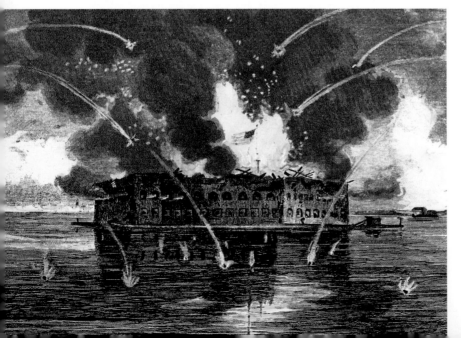

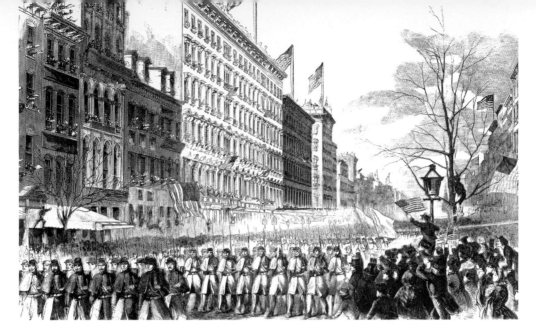
Volunteer soldiers helped strengthen the Union army.

Fort Sumter surrendered. Lincoln called on state **militias** to volunteer for federal service and help reclaim federal property. States on the border of the Union and Confederate territories were put in a difficult position. The Confederacy would consider it an attack if they joined their militias to the Union forces. These states refused Lincoln's request. Virginia, Tennessee, North Carolina, and Arkansas joined the Confederacy. The American Civil War had begun.

Slavery in the South

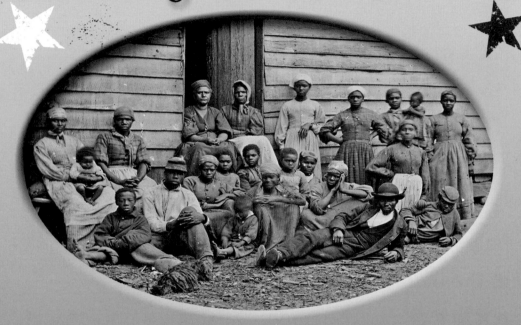

Millions of enslaved Africans were forced to work on southern plantations during the height of slavery in the United States. At one point, about 40 percent of all people living in the South were slaves. Slaves often lived and worked in poor conditions. They were treated harshly if they disobeyed their owners.

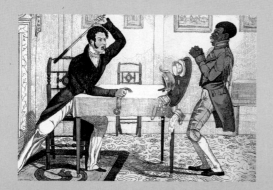

Resistance and Punishment

Some slaves defied their masters by working slowly, breaking tools, or refusing to work at all. Slaves were often whipped or tortured for this.

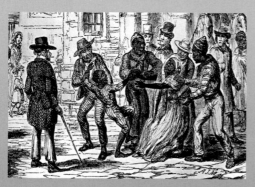

Destroyed Families

Slaves were bought and sold at their owners' will. Many slave families were separated. Owners sometimes did this to punish slaves.

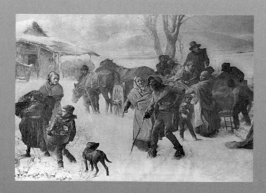

The Underground Railroad

Slaves often attempted to escape. Northerners often helped slaves escape to freedom in northern states or Canada. The routes were known as the Underground Railroad.

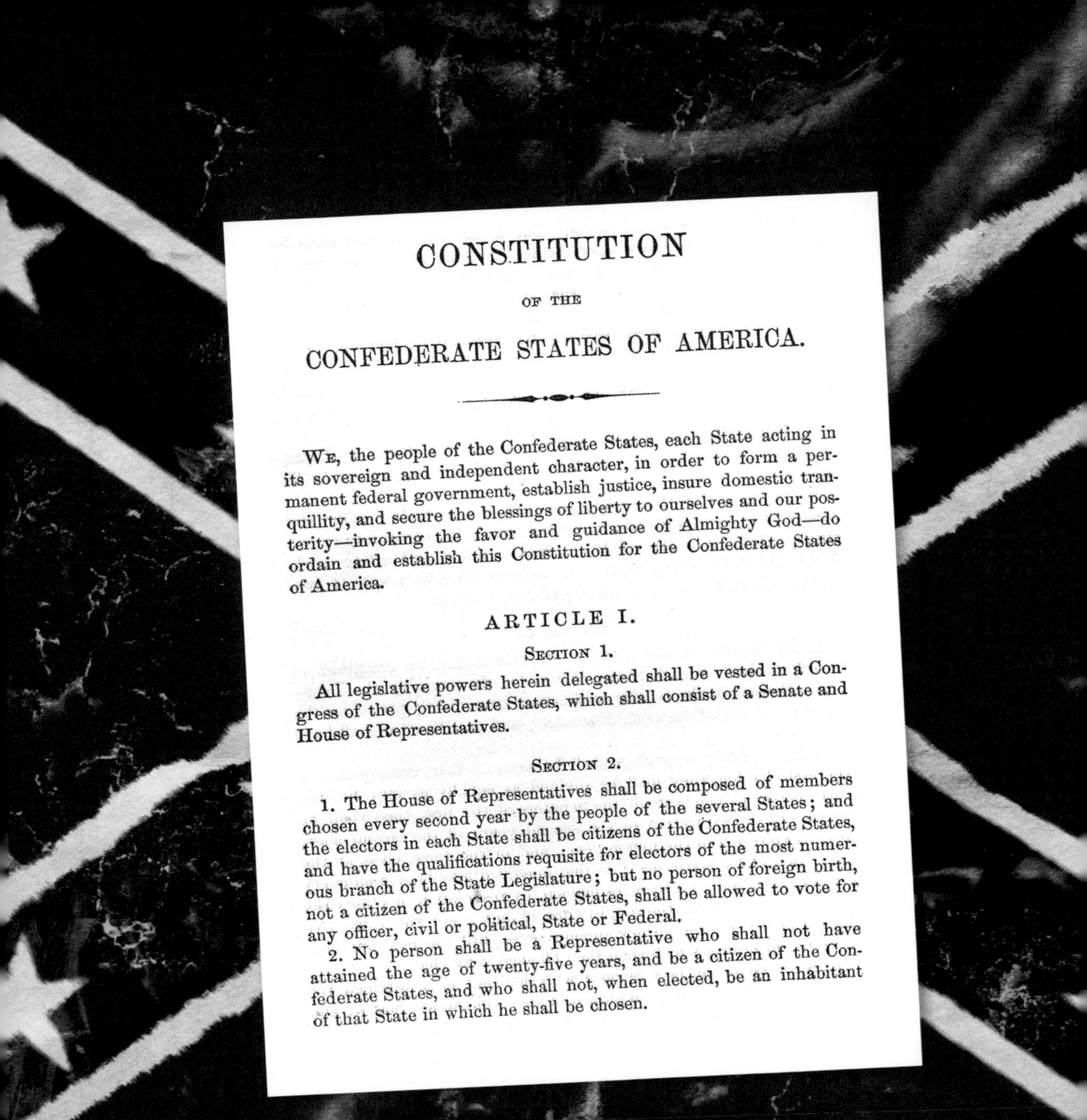

CONSTITUTION

OF THE

CONFEDERATE STATES OF AMERICA.

———————•◆•———————

WE, the people of the Confederate States, each State acting in its sovereign and independent character, in order to form a permanent federal government, establish justice, insure domestic tranquillity, and secure the blessings of liberty to ourselves and our posterity—invoking the favor and guidance of Almighty God—do ordain and establish this Constitution for the Confederate States of America.

ARTICLE I.

SECTION 1.

All legislative powers herein delegated shall be vested in a Congress of the Confederate States, which shall consist of a Senate and House of Representatives.

SECTION 2.

1. The House of Representatives shall be composed of members chosen every second year by the people of the several States; and the electors in each State shall be citizens of the Confederate States, and have the qualifications requisite for electors of the most numerous branch of the State Legislature; but no person of foreign birth, not a citizen of the Confederate States, shall be allowed to vote for any officer, civil or political, State or Federal.

2. No person shall be a Representative who shall not have attained the age of twenty-five years, and be a citizen of the Confederate States, and who shall not, when elected, be an inhabitant of that State in which he shall be chosen.

The Confederate Constitution was based mainly on the U.S. Constitution.

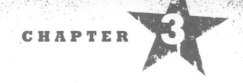

CHAPTER 3

The Confederate Government

The Confederacy had its own constitution. Slavery was upheld. Protective tariffs were forbidden. The Confederate Constitution also guaranteed the rights of all slave owners. Unlike the U.S. government, the Confederacy did not allow money raised from taxes in one state to be spent on improvements for a different state.

The Confederate Constitution was signed by 44 representatives from seven states.

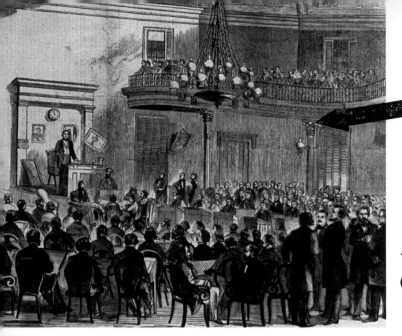

Howell Cobb, the president of the Confederate Congress, was a former U.S. Speaker of the House.

The Confederate Congress was very similar to the U.S. Congress.

The Confederate president would be elected to one six-year term. Reelection was not allowed. The Confederate Constitution also established a **legislature** with two houses. The Senate was made up of two senators from each of the 11 Confederate states. There were also two each from Kentucky and Missouri. These two states were not part of the Confederacy. But they both had populations that showed significant Confederate support.

The Confederate Congress had a House of Representatives with 109 members. It also contained a small number of Native American delegates. They were not allowed to vote. State legislatures chose senators, and voters elected the representatives. The Confederacy did not have a supreme court. It used a local court system instead. District judges and state courts continued to operate as they had before.

The first Confederate White House was located in Montgomery, Alabama.

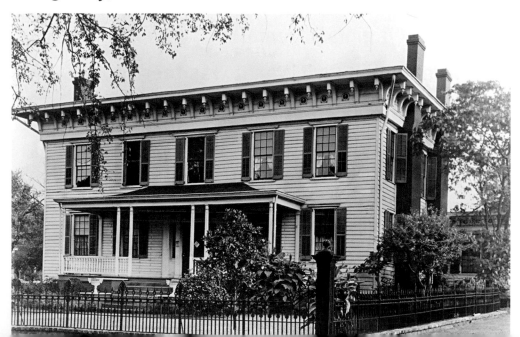

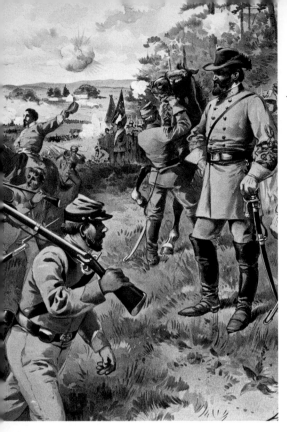

 Thomas "Stonewall" Jackson earned his nickname by holding back Union forces at the Battle of Bull Run in 1861.

A Capital in Motion

For a short time, the Confederate capital was located in Montgomery, Alabama. In May 1861, it was relocated to Richmond, Virginia. It remained there until the final week of the Civil War. It was then moved again to Danville, Virginia. The Confederacy maintained its own army, navy, and marines. These military forces were put to use almost immediately when the Civil War broke out shortly after the Confederacy formed.

A Shortage of Soldiers

By April 16, 1862, Confederate leaders had decided that it would be necessary to require all men between the ages of 18 and 35 to serve in the military. But **desertion** was a constant problem. Certain groups of people, such as planters, were excused from joining. The system became dishonest. Confederate states sometimes refused to supply troops. They used states' rights as an excuse.

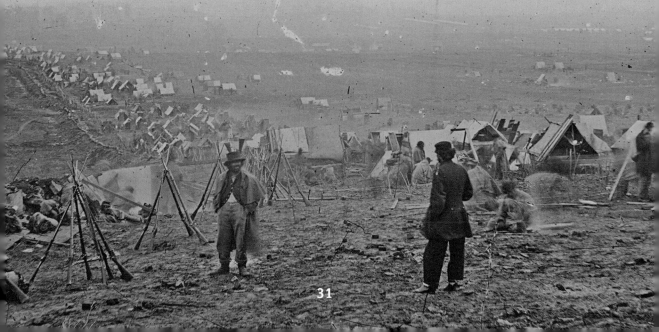

Diplomacy

The Confederacy printed its own paper money and had its own national flag. The Confederacy tried to win recognition and support throughout Europe for its war with the United States. Numerous European countries were sympathetic to the Confederacy. But President Lincoln warned Europe that support for the Confederacy meant war with the United States.

Like the U.S. flag, the Confederate national flag had a star for each state.

More stars were added to the Confederate flag as more states joined the Confederacy.

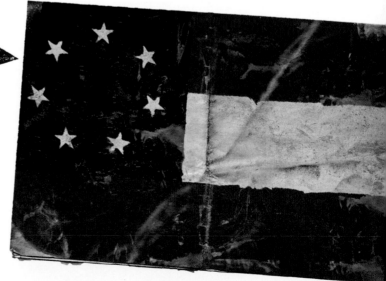

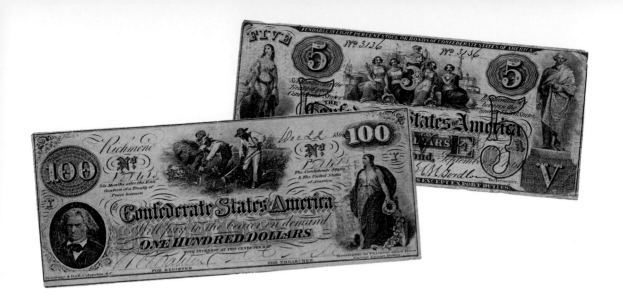

Some Confederate money featured pictures of slaves working in fields.

Inflation

Diplomacy was failing. The Confederacy applied economic pressure to Europe by slowing exports of cotton. But the Confederate war effort was doomed without the money that came from cotton sales. The Confederacy began printing large amounts of paper money to pay for its expenses. This caused severe **inflation**. The Confederate dollar had almost no value by the end of the war. The South's economy was badly damaged.

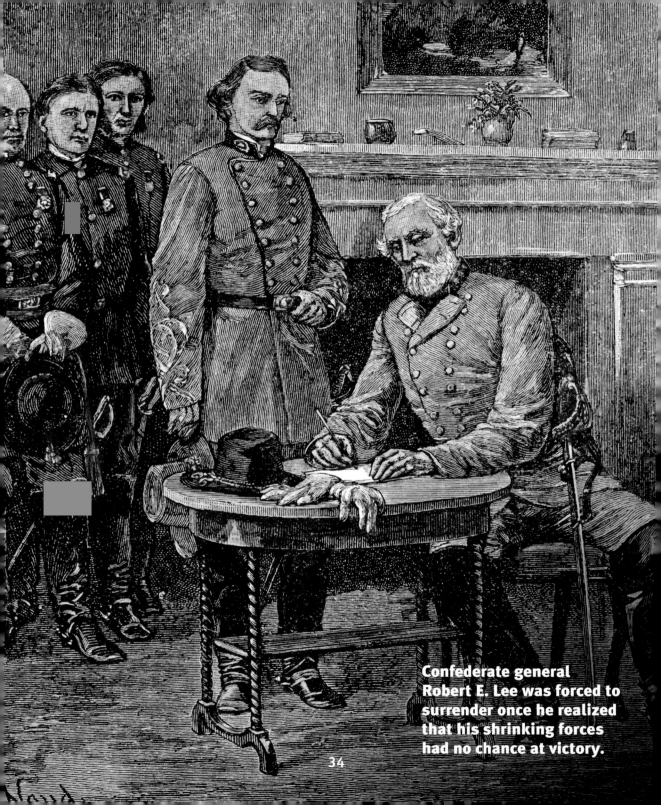

Confederate general
Robert E. Lee was forced to
surrender once he realized
that his shrinking forces
had no chance at victory.

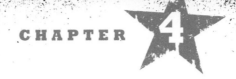

The End of an Era

Hundreds of thousands of lives on both sides were lost during the four years of fighting in the Civil War. The Confederacy had failed to gain recognition. Confederate general Robert E. Lee surrendered to Union general Ulysses S. Grant at Appomattox Court House in Virginia on April 9, 1865. This made victory a sure thing for the Union. But what exactly caused the Confederacy's defeat?

 Appomattox Court House became a national historic monument in 1940.

Economic Issues

The odds of winning the war were immediately against the Confederacy because of the Union's economic superiority. The Confederacy had the advantage of its enormous agricultural production. But the Northern states had more than twice the Confederacy's population and more than three times its wealth. Northern states also had a far more developed railroad system and much more manufacturing.

Timeline of the Confederacy

1828

The U.S. government places a high tariff on imported goods.

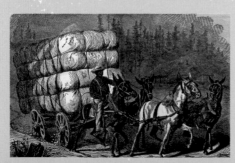

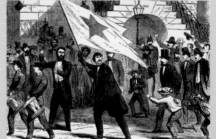

1860

South Carolina secedes from the Union.

The Confederacy also failed to defend its territory throughout the war. The Union forces attacked Southern territory and destroyed important resources. The Confederate forces hoped to convince the Union that the cost of war was too great to continue fighting. They believed that Union support for the war would disappear when Lincoln's term as president ended. These hopes were crushed when Lincoln was reelected in 1864.

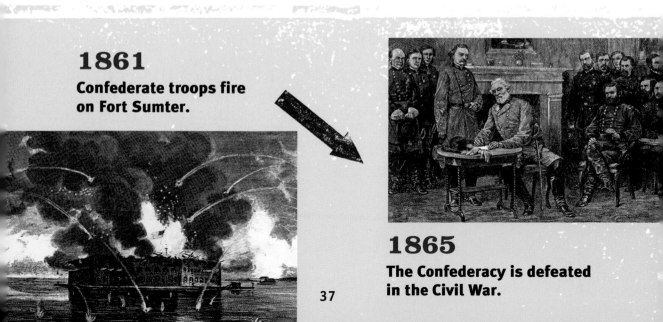

1861
Confederate troops fire on Fort Sumter.

1865
The Confederacy is defeated in the Civil War.

No Support From Europe

The Confederacy's failure to gain the support of France and Great Britain also contributed to its downfall. It came close to gaining Great Britain's help because of the two countries' economic importance

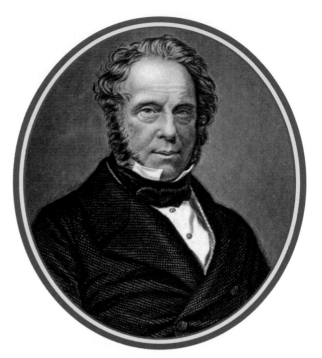

British prime minister Henry John Temple believed that Great Britain should stay neutral during the Civil War.

to one another. But Union diplomats were able to convince the Europeans to stay out of the war. This denied the Confederates valuable resources and military assistance.

Leadership Weakness?

Some historians believe that the Confederacy's biggest problem was a lack of good military leaders. Generals such as Stonewall Jackson and James Longstreet were excellent at leading smaller groups of soldiers. But they were unable to successfully manage the huge numbers of forces they commanded during the Civil War. General Robert E. Lee showed military genius and dynamic leadership. But this was not enough to carry the entire Confederate war effort.

Lee's father was a close friend of George Washington's.

Despite his considerable leadership skills, Robert E. Lee was not able to win the war.

Other historians point to disagreements between Confederate leaders as a major problem. Jefferson Davis was known for being stubborn. Vice President Stephens often disagreed with him publicly. Conflicts such as these may prevent any government from working smoothly. Confederate leaders did not make fast decisions when they were needed. They often argued over how to proceed.

Davis fled south from the capital when he heard of Lee's surrender at Appomattox.

Jefferson Davis did not have the leadership skills needed to run a new nation effectively.

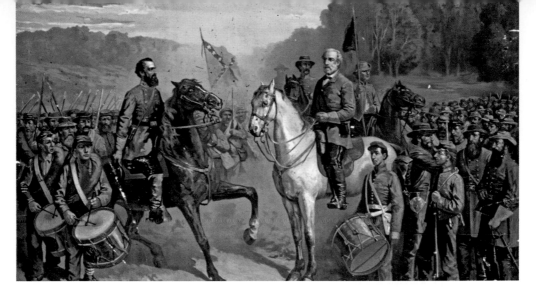

Confederate military leaders often had trouble getting their men to follow orders because of Southern belief in individualism.

Too Much Freedom

The Confederates' strong belief in individual freedom may have contributed to their defeat as well. Members of the Confederate military would sometimes refuse to follow orders from superior officers. Many saw Davis's decision to require military service as an attempt to destroy states' rights. The Confederacy lacked the two-party political system of the Union. This meant that few alternatives to Davis's policies were put forward.

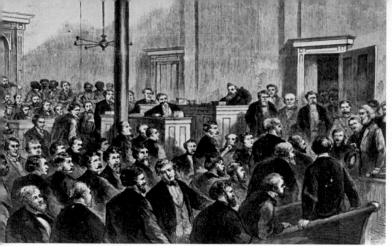

Davis received offers of free defense from multiple Northern lawyers.

Jefferson Davis never received a proper trial for his crimes.

After the War

The Confederate government officially ended on May 5, 1865. Five days later, Davis was captured, charged with treason (helping the enemy during war), and imprisoned. He was released after two years. The war was costly for both the Northern and Southern states. It took years to rebuild the bonds between them. There is still disagreement to this day about states' rights. But people have come to rely on political debate instead of secession to achieve their goals. ★

True Statistics

First state to secede from the Union: South Carolina

Number of Confederate states: 11

Confederate president's length of term: 6 years

Number of houses in Confederate legislature: 2

Number of men elected to Confederate House of Representatives: 109

Date of Confederate attack on Fort Sumter: April 12, 1861

Ages of men required to serve in Confederate military: 18 to 35

Years Civil War was fought: 1861 to 1865

Place where the South surrendered to the Union: Appomattox Court House, Virginia

Length of the Confederacy's existence: Less than 5 years

Did you find the truth?

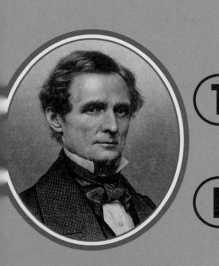

T The Confederate States of America were formed before President Abraham Lincoln took office.

F Confederate president Jefferson Davis was executed after the Civil War.

Resources

Books

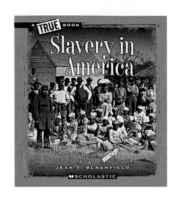

Aretha, David. *Jefferson Davis*. New York: Chelsea House, 2009.

Blashfield, Jean F. *Slavery in America*. New York: Children's Press, 2012.

Collins, Terry. *Robert E. Lee: The Story of the Great Confederate General*. Mankato, MN: Capstone Press, 2011.

Gillis, Jennifer Blizin. *The Confederate Soldier*. Minneapolis: Compass Point Books, 2007.

Grant, R. G. *Slavery: Real People and Their Stories of Enslavement*. New York: DK Publishing, 2009.

Olson, Kay Melchisedech. *The Terrible, Awful Civil War*. Mankato, MN: Capstone Press, 2010.

Somervill, Barbara A. *Women of the Confederacy*. Minneapolis: Compass Point Books, 2007.

Williams, Jean Kinney. *Jefferson Davis: President of the Confederacy*. Minneapolis: Compass Point Books, 2005.

Organizations and Web Sites

History.com — Jefferson Davis

www.history.com/topics/jefferson-davis

Learn more about the life and accomplishments of the only president of the Confederate States of America.

PBS — Map: The Confederate States of America

www.pbs.org/civilwar/war/map1.html

Check out a map of the Confederate states and read more about the Civil War.

Places to Visit

Appomattox Court House National Historical Park

Highway 24, PO Box 218
Appomattox, VA 24522
(434) 352-8987 ext. 26
www.nps.gov/apco/index.htm
Take a tour of the historic site where Confederate general Robert E. Lee surrendered to Union general Ulysses S. Grant.

Fort Sumter National Monument

1214 Middle Street
Sullivan's Island, SC 29482
(843) 883-3123
www.nps.gov/fosu/index.htm
Walk the grounds where the first shots of the Civil War were fired and view one of the best collections of 19th-century seacoast artillery anywhere in the United States.

Important Words

abolition (ab-uh-LIH-shuhn)—the official end of something

delegates (DEL-i-gitz)—people who represent other people at a meeting or in a legislature

desertion (di-ZUR-shuhn)—to run away from the army

diplomacy (duh-PLOH-muh-see)—establishing relations between different countries

economy (i-KON-uh-mee)—the way a country runs its industry, trade, and finance

federal (FED-ur-uhl)—a several states united under and controlled by one central power

inflation (in-FLAY-shuhn)—a general increase in prices

legislature (LEJ-is-lay-chur) —a group of people who have the power to make or change the laws of a country or state

militias (muh-LISH-uhz)—groups of people who are trained to fight but who aren't professional soldiers

nullification (nuh-lih-fih-KAY-shuhn)—to have canceled or made of no value

plantations (plan-TAY-shuhnz)—large farms found in warm climates

seceded (si-SEED-id)—withdrew formally from a group or an organization

tariff (TA-rif)—a tax on goods that are imported or exported

Index

Page numbers in **bold** indicate illustrations

About the Author

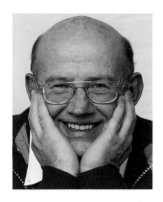

Peter Benoit is educated as a mathematician but has many other interests. He has taught and tutored high school and college students for many years, mostly in math and science. He also runs summer workshops for writers and students of literature. Mr. Benoit has also written more than 2,000 poems. His life has been one committed to learning. He lives in Greenwich, New York.